T0259407

Precision Medicine in Surgical Oncology

Editors

VIJAY P. KHATRI
NICHOLAS J. PETRELLI

SURGICAL ONCOLOGY
CLINICS OF NORTH AMERICA

www.surgonc.theclinics.com

Consulting Editor
TIMOTHY M. PAWLIK

January 2020 • Volume 29 • Number 1

ELSEVIER

1600 John F. Kennedy Boulevard • Suite 1800 • Philadelphia, Pennsylvania, 19103-2899

http://www.theclinics.com

SURGICAL ONCOLOGY CLINICS OF NORTH AMERICA Volume 29, Number 1
January 2020 ISSN 1055-3207, ISBN-13: 978-0-323-69737-8

Editor: John Vassallo (j.vassallo@elsevier.com)
Developmental Editor: Laura Kavanaugh

Surgical Oncology Clinics of North America (ISSN 1055-3207) is published quarterly by Elsevier Inc., 360 Park Avenue South, New York, NY 10010-1710. Months of publication are January, April, July, and October. Business and Editorial Offices: 1600 John F. Kennedy Blvd., Ste. 1800, Philadelphia, PA 19103-2899. Customer Service Office: 3251 Riverport Lane, Maryland Heights, MO 63043. Periodicals postage paid at New York, NY and additional mailing offices. Subscription prices are $309.00 per year (US individuals), $562.00 (US institutions) $100.00 (US student/resident), $352.00 (Canadian individuals), $711.00 (Canadian institutions), $100.00 (Canadian student/resident), $422.00 (foreign individuals), $711.00 (foreign institutions), and $205.00 (foreign student/resident). Foreign air speed delivery is included in all *Clinics* subscription prices. All prices are subject to change without notice. **POSTMASTER**: Send address changes to *Surgical Oncology Clinics of North America,* Elsevier Health Science Division, Subscription Customer Service, 3251 Riverport Lane, Maryland Heights, MO 63043. **Customer Service: 1-800-654-2452 (US and Canada). 314-447-8871 (outside US and Canada). Fax: 314-447-8029. E-mail: journalscustomerservice-usa@elsevier.com (for print support); journalsonline support-usa@elsevier.com (for online support).**

Reprints. For copies of 100 or more, of articles in this publication, please contact the Commercial Reprints Department, Elsevier Inc., 360 Park Avenue South, New York, New York 10010-1710. Tel. 212-633-3874; Fax: 212-633-3820; E-mail: reprints@elsevier.com.

Surgical Oncology Clinics of North America is covered in *MEDLINE/PubMed (Index Medicus)* and *EMBASE/ Excerpta Medica, Current Contents/Clinical Medicine, and ISI/BIOMED.*

Contributors

CONSULTING EDITOR

TIMOTHY M. PAWLIK, MD, MPH, MTS, PhD, FACS, FRACS (Hon)
Professor and Chair, Department of Surgery, The Urban Meyer III and Shelley Meyer Chair for Cancer Research, Professor of Surgery, Oncology, Health Services Management and Policy, Surgeon-in-Chief, The Ohio State University, Wexner Medical Center, Columbus, Ohio, USA

EDITORS

VIJAY P. KHATRI, MBChB, MBA, FACS
Professor of Oncology, Department of Surgery, Assistant Dean of Faculty Affairs, California Northstate University College of Medicine, Elk Grove, California, USA

NICHOLAS J. PETRELLI, MD, FACS
Bank of America Endowed Medical Director, Department of Surgery, Helen F. Graham Cancer Center and Research Institute, Christiana Care Health System, Newark, Delaware, USA; Professor, Department of Surgery, Thomas Jefferson University, Philadelphia, Pennsylvania, USA

AUTHORS

KIMBERLY ADERHOLD, DO
Thomas Jefferson University Hospital–Sidney Kimmel Cancer Center, Philadelphia, Pennsylvania, USA

PHILIPPE ARMAND, MD, PhD
Medical Oncology, Associate Professor of Medicine, Harvard Medical School, Dana-Farber Cancer Institute, Boston, Massachusetts, USA

ROXANNE BAVARIAN, DMD
Division of Oral Medicine and Dentistry, Brigham and Women's Hospital, Harvard School of Dental Medicine, Boston, Massachusetts, USA

JOSEPH BENNETT, MD, FACS
Department of Surgery, Christiana Care Health System, Newark, Delaware, USA

ADAM C. BERGER, MD, FACS
Professor of Surgery and Chief of Melanoma and Soft Tissue Oncology, Rutgers Cancer Institute of New Jersey, New Brunswick, New Jersey, USA

ADITI BHATTACHARYA, BDS, MDS, PhD
Assistant Professor, Department of Oral and Maxillofacial Surgery, NYU College of Dentistry, New York, New York, USA

BRITTANY N. BURTON, MHS
Medical Student, School of Medicine, University of California, San Diego, San Diego, California, USA

MARCO CARBONE, MD, PhD
Division of Gastroenterology and Hepatology, Department of Medicine and Surgery, University of Milan Bicocca, Milan, Italy; Academic Department of Medical Genetics, University of Cambridge, Cambridge, United Kingdom

LOGAN COREY, MD
Ob/Gyn Resident, Department of Obstetrics and Gynecology, Ochsner Clinic Foundation, New Orleans, Louisiana, USA

LAURA CRISTOFERI, MD
Division of Gastroenterology and Hepatology, Department of Medicine and Surgery, University of Milan Bicocca, Milan, Italy

JENNIFER L. CROMBIE, MD
Medical Oncology, Instructor of Medicine, Harvard Medical School, Dana-Farber Cancer Institute, Boston, Massachusetts, USA

SHIBANDRI DAS, MD
Surgical Resident, University Hospitals Cleveland Medical Center, MetroHealth Hospitals, Louis Stokes Veterans Administration Hospital, Case Western Reserve University, Cleveland, Ohio, USA

DEBORAH B. DOROSHOW, MD, PhD
Assistant Professor of Medicine, Department of Medicine and Cancer Center, Icahn School of Medicine at Mount Sinai, New York, New York, USA

JAMES H. DOROSHOW, MD
Director, Division of Cancer Treatment and Diagnosis, National Cancer Institute, National Institutes of Health, Bethesda, Maryland, USA

RODNEY A. GABRIEL, MD, MAS
Chief, Division of Regional Anesthesia and Acute Pain, Assistant Clinical Professor, Department of Anesthesiology, Department of Medicine, Division of Biomedical Informatics, University of California, San Diego, San Diego, California, USA

IAN GREENWALT, MD
Chief Surgical Resident, University Hospitals Cleveland Medical Center, MetroHealth Hospitals, Louis Stokes Veterans Administration Hospital, Case Western Reserve University, Cleveland, Ohio, USA

PIETRO INVERNIZZI, MD, PhD
Division of Gastroenterology and Hepatology, Department of Medicine and Surgery, University of Milan Bicocca, Milan, Italy

VIJAY P. KHATRI, MBChB, MBA, FACS
Professor of Oncology, Department of Surgery, Assistant Dean of Faculty Affairs, California Northstate University College of Medicine, Elk Grove, California, USA

JOSEPH LEONG, BS
Department of Surgery, California Northstate University College of Medicine, Elk Grove, California, USA

SHOSHANA LEVI, MD
Department of Surgery, Christiana Care Health System, Newark, Delaware, USA

BENJAMIN D. LI, MD, MBA, FACS
MetroHealth Cancer Center Director, MetroHealth System, Edward Mansour Professor of Surgical Oncology, Case Western Reserve University, Cancer Care Pavilion, Cleveland, Ohio, USA

CHIA-CHENG LI, DDS, DMSc
Instructor of Oral Medicine, Infection, and Immunity, Department of Oral Medicine, Infection, and Immunity, Harvard School of Dental Medicine, Boston, Massachusetts, USA

GREGORY A. MASTERS, MD, FACP, FASCO
Attending Physician, Helen F. Graham Cancer Center and Research Institute, Newark, Delaware, USA; Associate Professor, Thomas Jefferson University Medical School, , Philadelphia, Pennsylvania, USA

GEORGE MELLS, MRCP, PhD
Academic Department of Medical Genetics, University of Cambridge, Cambridge, United Kingdom

ALESSANDRA NARDI, PhD
Department of Mathematics, Tor Vergata University of Rome, Rome, Italy

D. WILLIAMS PARSONS, MD, PhD
Section of Hematology/Oncology, Department of Pediatrics, Baylor College of Medicine, Texas Children's Hospital, Houston, Texas, USA

NICHOLAS J. PETRELLI, MD, FACS
Bank of America Endowed Medical Director, Department of Surgery, Helen F. Graham Cancer Center and Research Institute, Christiana Care Health System, Newark, Delaware, USA; Professor, Department of Surgery, Thomas Jefferson University, Philadelphia, Pennsylvania, USA

SANGEETHA PRABHAKARAN, MD, FACS
Assistant Professor of Surgery, Division of Surgical Oncology, Department of Surgery, University of New Mexico, Albuquerque, New Mexico, USA

NITA L. SEIBEL, MD
Division of Cancer Treatment and Diagnosis, Clinical Investigations Branch, National Cancer Institute, Rockville, Maryland, USA

DHAVAL R. SHAH, MBBS, MD
Attending Physician, Helen F. Graham Cancer Center and Research Institute, Newark, Delaware, USA

ZHEN SHEN, PhD
Harvard School of Dental Medicine, Boston, Massachusetts, USA

RICHARD D. URMAN, MD, MBA, FASA
Associate Professor, Department of Anesthesiology, Perioperative and Pain Medicine, Harvard Medical School, Brigham and Women's Hospital, Boston, Massachusetts, USA

ANA VALENTE, MD
Ob/Gyn Resident, Department of Obstetrics and Gynecology, Ochsner Clinic Foundation, New Orleans, Louisiana, USA

KIEUHOA T. VO, MD, MAS
Department of Pediatrics, University of California San Francisco School of Medicine, Benioff Children's Hospital, San Francisco, California, USA

KATRINA WADE, MD
Gynecologic Oncologist, Department of Gynecologic Oncology, Ochsner Clinic Foundation, New Orleans, Louisiana, USA

RUTH S. WATERMAN, MD, MSc
Chair, Associate Clinical Professor, Department of Anesthesiology, University of California, San Diego, San Diego, California, USA

MELISSA WILSON, MD, PhD
Associate Professor, Sidney Kimmel Medical College, Philadelphia, Pennsylvania, USA

FAN YANG, DDS, PhD
Harvard School of Dental Medicine, Boston, Massachusetts, USA

NORAH ZAZA, BA
Medical Student, Case Western Reserve University, Cleveland, Ohio, USA

Contents

> Translational and clinical research advances have unveiled extensive cancer tumor cell heterogenicity. New understanding has prompted the practice-changing treatment of each cancer specific to its unique genetic construct. Among the earliest applications of this model was melanoma treatment. Survival rates increased significantly, with improvement each year. Genetic profiling allows further lesion classification, resulting in more personalized follow-up and treatment plans. Gene expression profiling allows the identification of specific mutations to direct targeted therapy and provides invaluable prognostic data. This article reviews the newest and most up-to-date advances in precision medicine within melanoma practice.

> Lung cancer remains second most common cancer in men and women in the United States. More than 50% of patients are diagnosed in the advanced stage. Traditionally, chemotherapy has been the backbone of management of stage IV lung cancer. A better understanding of the molecular pathogenesis has led to rapid development of targeted therapy and immunotherapy. This has led to significant improvement in survival of patients with lung cancer stages III to IV. These drugs are being studied in early stage lung cancer. Several trials are ongoing to improve the survival and quality of life of our patients.

> This article reviews advances in precision medicine for colorectal carcinoma that have influenced screening and treatment, and potentially prevention. Advances in molecular techniques have made it possible for better patient selection for therapies; therefore, mutational analysis should be performed at diagnosis to guide treatment. Future efforts should focus on validating these treatments in specific subgroups and on understanding the mechanisms of resistance to therapies to enable treatment optimization, promote efficacy, and reduce treatment costs and toxicities.

opioids, nonopioid analgesics, sedatives, β-blockers, antiemetics, and anticoagulants) used in the perioperative process and the challenges of integrating PGx into a health care system and relevant workflows.

Individualizing Care: Management Beyond Medical Therapy

Laura Cristoferi, Alessandra Nardi, Pietro Invernizzi, George Mells, and Marco Carbone

> The evolving research landscape, with advances in the omics technologies, availability of large-scale patient cohorts, and forthcoming availability of novel drugs in primary biliary cholangitis (PBC), is creating a unique opportunity for developing a precision medicine (PM) program. PM has potential to change the paradigm of management. Diagnostic work-up of PBC patients may include information on genetic variants and molecular signature to define a particular subtype of disease and provide an estimate of treatment response and survival. To reach this point, specific interventions, such as sequencing more genomes, creating bigger biobanks, and linking biological information to health data, are needed.

Personalized Medicine in Gynecologic Cancer: Fact or Fiction?

Logan Corey, Ana Valente, and Katrina Wade

> Personalized medicine in gynecologic oncology is an evolving field. In recent years, tumor profiling and large databases such as TCGA and NCI-Match have provided us with enormous amounts of molecular data. Several therapies that capitalize on novel genetic and immune discoveries including VEGF inhibitors, PARP inhibitors, and cancer vaccinations are discussed in this article. Additionally, we have seen direct to consumer marketing play an important role in cancer care and prevention as patients have increased ability to access genetic testing. This presents a unique challenge to gynecologic oncology providers as we learn to navigate the world of personalized medicine.

Diffuse Large B-Cell Lymphoma and High-Grade B-Cell Lymphoma: Genetic Classification and Its Implications for Prognosis and Treatment

Jennifer L. Crombie and Philippe Armand

> Diffuse large B-cell lymphoma (DLBCL), the most common subtype of non-Hodgkin lymphoma, is characterized by both clinical and molecular heterogeneity. Despite efforts to tailor therapy for individual patients, treatment remains uniform and a subset of patients have poor outcomes. The past decade has witnessed a dramatic expansion of our understanding of the genomic underpinnings of this disease, especially with the application of next-generation sequencing. In this review, the authors highlight the current genomic landscape of DLBCL and how this information provides a potential molecular framework for precision medicine-based strategies in this disease.

Oral Cancer: Genetics and the Role of Precision Medicine

Chia-Cheng Li, Zhen Shen, Roxanne Bavarian, Fan Yang, and Aditi Bhattacharya

> Oral squamous cell carcinoma (OSCC) is one of the leading cancers in the world. OSCC patients are managed with surgery and/or chemoradiation.

Prognoses and survival rates are dismal, however, and have not improved for more than 20 years. Recently, the concept of precision medicine was introduced, and the introduction of targeted therapeutics demonstrated promising outcomes. This article reviews the current understanding of initiation, progression, and metastasis of OSCC from both genetic and epigenetic perspectives. In addition, the applications and integration of omics technologies in biomarker discovery and drug development for treating OSCC are reviewed.

SURGICAL ONCOLOGY
CLINICS OF NORTH AMERICA

SERIES OF RELATED INTEREST

Surgical Clinics of North America
http://www.surgical.theclinics.com
Thoracic Surgery Clinics
http://www.thoracic.theclinics.com
Advances in Surgery
http://www.advancessurgery.com

THE CLINICS ARE AVAILABLE ONLINE!
Access your subscription at:
www.theclinics.com

SURGICAL ONCOLOGY
CLINICS OF NORTH AMERICA

FORTHCOMING ISSUES

April 2020
Management of GI and Pancreatic
Neuroendocrine Tumors
James R. Howe, Editor

July 2020
Melanoma
Keith Delman, Michael Lowe, Editors

RECENT ISSUES

October 2019
Biliary Tract and Primary Liver Tumors
T. Clark Gamblin, Editor

July 2019
Immunotherapy for Solid Malignancies
Alfred E. Chang, Editor

SERIES OF RELATED INTEREST

Surgical Clinics of North America
http://www.surgical.theclinics.com
Thoracic Surgery Clinics
http://www.thoracic.theclinics.com
Advances in Surgery
http://www.advancessurgery.com

THE CLINICS ARE AVAILABLE ONLINE!
Access your subscription at:
www.theclinics.com

Foreword

Precision Medicine in Surgical Oncology

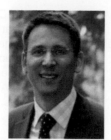

Timothy M. Pawlik, MD, MPH, MTS, PhD, FACS, FRACS (Hon)
Consulting Editor

This issue of the *Surgical Oncology Clinics of North America* is devoted to covering the important emerging topic of Precision Medicine in Surgical Oncology. As surgeons, it is critical that we integrate new knowledge about precision medicine into the diagnosis and surgical management of patients with cancer. The guest editors are Dr Vijay Khatri and Dr Nicholas Petrelli. Both Drs Khatri and Petrelli are recognized leaders in surgery with particular expertise in emerging innovative therapies for patients with cancer. Dr Khatri is Assistant Dean of Faculty Affairs, Professor of Surgery and Oncology at California Northstate University College of Medicine. Dr Khatri is an experienced academic surgical oncologist, as well as a physician executive with experience in cancer surgery. In addition, Dr Khatri serves as Editor-in-Chief of *Surgical Oncology*, which is a leading journal in the field. Dr Petrelli is a nationally recognized expert on colorectal cancer, and the endowed medical director of the Graham Cancer Center within the Christiana Care Health System. Dr Petrelli has conducted substantial research into the genetics of colorectal cancer and coauthored more than 300 articles in peer-reviewed journals. Both Drs Khatri and Petrelli have immense expertise in the treatment of patients with cancer and have played pivotal roles in advancing the field of surgical oncology. As such, Drs Khatri and Petrelli are ideally suited to be the guest editors of this important issue of the *Surgical Oncology Clinics of North America*.

The issue covers a number of important topics, including the application of precision medicine to a wide array of different malignancies, including melanoma, lung, colon cancers, as well as pediatric oncology. The issue also includes perspectives on other significant subjects, such as genomics testing and personalized medicine in the preoperative setting, individualizing patient care beyond medical therapy, as well as genomics and the history of precision oncology. To accomplish such a far-reaching and comprehensive state-of-the-art review on this wide range of topics, Drs Khatri and Petrelli engaged an amazing group of authors who are leaders in their respective fields.

Surg Oncol Clin N Am 29 (2020) xiii–xiv
https://doi.org/10.1016/j.soc.2019.09.002
1055-3207/20/© 2019 Published by Elsevier Inc.

surgonc.theclinics.com

As you will see for yourself in reading this issue, Drs Khatri and Petrelli and the authors strongly demonstrate the importance and relevance of precision medicine as it relates to surgical oncology. In turn, I believe that the knowledge contained in this issue of *Surgical Oncology Clinics of North America* will serve to help surgical oncologists in the care of their patients. I would like to thank Drs Khatri and Petrelli and all the contributing authors for an excellent issue of the *Surgical Oncology Clinics of North America* that tackles such an important topic.

Timothy M. Pawlik, MD, MPH, MTS, PhD, FACS, FRACS (Hon)
Department of Surgery
Oncology and Health Services Management and Policy
The Ohio State University
Wexner Medical Center
395 West 12th Avenue, Suite 670
Columbus, OH 43210, USA

E-mail address:
tim.pawlik@osumc.edu

Preface

Precision Medicine

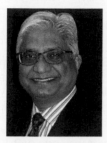
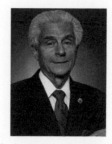

Vijay P. Khatri, MBChB, MBA, FACS   Nicholas J. Petrelli, MD, FACS
Editors

If the definition of precision medicine is looked up just about anywhere, in so many words it will be described as medical care to optimize efficiency or therapeutic benefit for particular groups of patients, especially by using genetic or molecular profiling. There is no question that we are in the era of precision medicine as demonstrated by the variety of topics dedicated to precision medicine in cancer treatment and prognosis in this issue of the *Surgical Oncology Clinics of North America*. It is an era that allows oncologists to accurately predict which treatment strategy will be effective for a particular cancer. To a certain extent, we have left behind the era of "one-size-fits-all approach," where patients are treated as a group without consideration for differences between individuals and their genetic profiles.

Although precision medicine, especially in cancer care, is new, the concept itself is not. This is demonstrated in any individual who needs a blood transfusion who is not given blood from any donor. Blood typing is necessary to match the individual receiving the transfusion so that any complications are avoided or certainly the risk of complications is reduced. This is also true if an individual has an allergy where they will get tested to determine exactly what the individual is allergic to. In 2016, the President's budget included investments in the emerging field of precision medicine, taking into account individual differences in people's environments, lifestyles, and genes.

The authors in this issue of the *Surgical Oncology Clinics of North America* give their perspective on the role of precision medicine in different cancer sites with not only

Surg Oncol Clin N Am 29 (2020) xv–xvi
https://doi.org/10.1016/j.soc.2019.10.001
1055-3207/20/© 2019 Published by Elsevier Inc.

where we are today but also the potential for the future. We congratulate all the authors for their contributions to this issue of the *Surgical Oncology Clinics of North America*.

Vijay P. Khatri, MBChB, MBA, FACS
California Northstate University
College of Medicine
Elk Grove, CA 95757, USA

Nicholas J. Petrelli, MD, FACS
Helen F. Graham Cancer Center &
Research Institute
Christiana Care Health System
Newark, DE 19713, USA

E-mail addresses:
vijay.khatri@cnsu.edu (V.P. Khatri)
NPetrelli@Christianacare.org (N.J. Petrelli)

Precision Medicine in the Treatment of Melanoma

Kimberly Aderhold, DO[a], Melissa Wilson, MD, PhD[a], Adam C. Berger, MD[c],*,
Shoshana Levi, MD[b], Joseph Bennett, MD[b]

KEYWORDS

- Melanoma • Precision medicine • Immunotherapy • Driver mutations • Oncogene
- Gene-expression • DecisionDx-melanoma

KEY POINTS

- There are a multitude of possible mutations across tumor genes with varying frequencies. Next-generation sequencing analyzes the tumor cells for all present mutations instead of sequential testing as was standard practice in years past.
- Precision medicine strategies targeting *BRAF*-V600 E/K mutations, with consequent suppression of the mitogen-activated protein kinase signaling pathway, have shown survival benefit in both the adjuvant and metastatic settings.
- MEK inhibitors have shown a small but significant progression-free survival advantage after failure of immunotherapy in *NRAS*-mutant melanoma.
- Immunotherapy with programmed death 1 and/or CTLA-4 inhibition has demonstrated substantial survival advantages in advanced resectable and unresectable melanomas.
- Gene expression profiling may influence postsurgical management by allowing more accurate risk stratification and, hence, more fitting follow-up and diagnostic testing.

Precision treatment of melanoma is rapidly evolving. Before the concept of precision medicine, the treatment of melanoma was limited to dacarbazine and interleukin-2 (IL-2), which achieved only a disappointingly small benefit in few patients with either therapy.[1] Now, however, profoundly more effective treatment options have been discovered that target actionable tumor-specific genetic mutations, including *BRAF*-V600 E/K driver mutations, *NRAS*, and *KIT* oncogenes, as well as immunotherapy with programmed death 1 (PD-1) and CTLA-4 inhibition. Often, these mutations are mutually

Disclosure Statement: Dr A.C. Berger has received honoraria from Castle Biosciences and Cardinal Health for consulting and speaker's bureau. Dr M. Wilson has received honoraria from BMS and Array Biopharma for advisory boards. The rest of the authors have nothing to disclose.
[a] Sidney Kimmel Medical College, Department of Medical Oncology, 1025 Walnut Street, Suite 700, Philadelphia, PA 19107, USA; [b] Department of Surgery, Christiana Care Health System, 4701 Ogletown Stanton Road, Newark, DE 19713, USA; [c] Rutgers Cancer Institute of New Jersey, 195 Little Albany Street, Room 3005, New Brunswick, NJ 08903, USA
* Corresponding author.
E-mail address: adam.berger@rutgers.edu

exclusive, usually only 1 mutation is found in a given tumor sample. Next-generation sequencing (NGS) testing has been instrumental in helping to identify large spans of tumor-specific genetic profiles that allow the opportunity to individualize each patient's treatment regimen based on the molecular biology of the tumor cells.

TARGETING BRAF AND MEK

The most common mutation found in melanoma is the *BRAF* driver mutation, with more than 90% of these mutations located at codon 600, termed *BRAF* V600 mutations. Those 10% of mutations not located at codon 600 are referred to as non-V600 *BRAF* mutations and are seen less frequently in melanoma. Additional non-V600 mutations are found in other tumor types, including lung and thyroid cancers.

Within *BRAF* V600 mutations, oncogenic driver mutations *BRAF*-V600 E and *BRAF*-V600 K are by far the most common subtypes in melanoma, having been identified in 40% to 60% of cutaneous melanomas.[2] These mutations within the mitogen-activated protein kinase (MAPK) signaling pathway, along with other pathway aberrations, including the MEK escape mechanisms and *NRAS* mutations, induce constitutive activation of the cell cycle, driving uncontrolled tumor proliferation. Suppression of these signaling pathways has been shown to be an effective strategy in the treatment of melanomas harboring these mutations. Furthermore, the upregulation of MEK 1/2 has been shown to be a prominent escape mechanism, leading to the use of combination therapy with BRAF and MEK inhibition.

BRAF inhibitors, such as dabrafenib and vemurafenib, have demonstrated a survival advantage as both monotherapy and in combination with the MEK inhibitor trametinib in both resectable and unresectable or metastatic melanomas.[3–5] The landmark BRIM-3, and BRIM-8, and coBRIM trials were the first to show the safety and efficacy of using vemurafenib to treat melanomas with *BRAF* V600 E and V600 E mutations.[3,6,7] Extended overall survival (OS) analysis published in 2017 on the 675 subjects studied in the phase III BRIM-3 clinical trial showed that vemurafenib continued to be associated with an improved median OS of 13.6 months versus 9.7 months with dacarbazine in subjects with untreated unresectable stage III or IV melanoma.[7,8]

Data from the breakthrough phase II and phase III clinical trials, BREAK-2 and BREAK-3, conducted in 2012 were the first to demonstrate a safe and effective progression-free survival (PFS) and an OS advantage with dabrafenib monotherapy.[9,10] The 5-year landmark analysis performed in 2017 of the phase III BREAK-3 trial described by Chapman and colleagues[11] showed sustainable and significant 5-year PFS (12% vs 3%) and OS (24% vs 22%) rates with single-agent dabrafenib compared with dacarbazine. A subset of subjects received CTLA-4 (24% vs 24%) and/or PD-1 (8% vs 2%) inhibitors after progression. Thirty-one percent versus 17% did not receive any therapy after long-term follow-up.

Furthermore, a phase III clinical trial conducted in 2015 by Robert and colleagues[5] showed that combination dabrafenib and trametinib had a superior OS rate (72% vs 65%) and PFS (11.4 months vs 7.3 months) when compared with vemurafenib alone in the metastatic setting. Similar results were seen in the metastatic setting in 2018 by Dummer and colleagues,[12] showing that the BRAF inhibitor encorafenib in combination with the MEK inhibitor binimetinib had a longer PFS of 14.9 months compared with 7.3 months with vemurafenib alone.

In adjuvant stage III and resected stage IV disease, the phase III clinical trial performed by Long and colleagues[4] in 2017 showed that combination BRAF and MEK inhibition had a superior 3-year relapse-free survival rate (58% vs 39%) and OS rate (86% vs 77%) compared with placebo. In 2018, a phase III clinical trial by Maio and colleagues[3] investigated the disease-free survival (DFS) of single-agent vemurafenib compared with placebo in 2 different cohorts. Cohort 1 included stage IIC, IIIA, and IIIB subjects with resectable disease, but the endpoint of median DFS was not reached. Cohort 2 studied stage IIIC resected disease and found a superior DFS of 23.1 months versus 15.4 months with placebo.

TARGETING NRAS

NRAS oncogenic mutations are seen in 15% to 20% of melanomas, and this distinct cohort of melanomas portend a poor prognosis.[13] Melanomas harboring this mutation tend to have more aggressive clinical and pathologic features, including increased mitotic activity, deeper depth of the lesion, and increased rates of nodal metastasis. The mutant allele varies within NRAS driver mutations. It is often found on codon Q61 (NRAS Q61) or less commonly on codons G12 and G13 (NRAS G12 and NRAS G13). Although all are considered activating point mutations, they affect the NRAS protein in different ways, leading to different clinical courses.[14]

Owing to the aggressive nature of NRAS mutant melanomas, investigation into potential therapeutic agents to target this oncogene has been of interest in the academic community. Preclinical models showed promising tumor response with first-generation MEK inhibitors to treat NRAS mutant melanomas. However, several of these trials did not show meaningful efficacy on further investigation.[13] These trials showed significant adverse events, namely ocular and neurologic symptoms that precluded further development of first-generation MEK inhibitors.

Newer second-generation MEK inhibitors subsequently were developed showing more tumor inhibition in preclinical models along with a tolerable safety profile. The first of these was selumetinib. A phase I study of 11 subjects with NRAS-mutant melanoma showed only partial response in 1 subject, and stable disease in 7 others. A subsequent phase II trial comparing selumetinib with temozolomide in NRAS-unselected subjects and BRAF-WT melanomas showed either equivalent or inferior response rates for selumetinib (5.8% vs 9.7%), as well as no benefit in PFS.[15] A second phase II study investigated selumetinib with or without dacarbazine in BRAF-WT melanomas but found similarly disappointing responses despite PFS being minimally prolonged (5.6 vs 3.0 months).[16]

Owing to the less than ideal results of selumetinib, development of third-generation MEK inhibitors led to even more promising results because focus shifted to NRAS-mutant melanomas. Dummer and colleagues[17] compared the third-generation MEK inhibitor binimetinib with standard-of-care dacarbazine in advanced or unresectable stage IIIC or IV NRAS-mutant melanomas. The study showed that binimetinib had a small but statistically significant superior median PFS of 2.8 months with binimetinib versus 1.5 months with dacarbazine. The small suboptimal response rates of third-generation MEK inhibitors led to consideration of combination strategies. Combinations of MEK inhibitors with CDK 4/6 inhibitors, RAF, and drugs targeting the EGFR/PI3K pathway have been considered in clinical trials.[14]

TARGETING KIT

Identification of the KIT oncogene led to multiple clinical trials studying transmembrane receptor tyrosine kinase as a target in the treatment of melanoma.[1] Binding of the KIT ligand results in activation of multiple downstream signaling pathways, including MAPK, JAK/STAT, and PI3K. Thus, the hypothesis evolved that targeting this mutation may provide an additional target for treatment of melanoma with the tyrosine kinase inhibitor imatinib.

Although several trials have shown efficacy of imatinib in treating melanomas harboring the KIT mutation, not all KIT mutations are sensitive to imatinib. As with NRAS and BRAF mutations, KIT mutations can vary widely over the genetic coding region, suggesting that not all mutations are equivalent functionally. There is some suggestion that certain mutations may represent passenger mutations instead of driver mutations. Demonstrating this concept, in the trial held by Guo and colleagues,[18] 9 of the 10 subjects who exhibited a response to imatinib had either exon 11 or 13 mutations, whereas there was only 1 of 3 subjects with KIT amplification who showed a response. This suggests that more specific molecular selection is necessary for effective targeted treatment with KIT inhibition.

Further defining the concept of more specific allelic selection when using imatinib to treat KIT mutant melanomas, 3 phase II studies between 2005 to 2008 revealed negative results, suggesting no benefit from KIT inhibition in metastatic melanoma. However, these studies were performed in molecularly unselected subject populations, and only 1 subject with acral melanoma from the 3 studies had a durable near-complete response. Interestingly, this subject had a splice site KIT mutation on exon 15.

Subsequent phase II clinical trials studying imatinib in molecularly selected advanced melanoma showed a small but significant efficacy in a subset of subjects who received imatinib. Carvajal and colleagues[19] showed significant clinical responses in 25 subjects with advanced melanoma, demonstrating an overall durable response rate for imatinib at 16% with a median time to progression of 12 weeks and a median OS of 46.3 weeks in a subset of subjects harboring primary KIT mutations. Similar findings were seen by Guo and colleagues,[18] who studied 43 subjects with advanced melanoma harboring KIT mutations and found an overall response rate of 23.3%, with a median PFS of 9 months and an OS of 15 months in those subjects who achieved a partial response or stable disease. Nine of the 10 subjects who achieved a partial response harbored KIT mutations on exon 11 or 13.

IMMUNOTHERAPY

Immunotherapy has revolutionized the treatment of melanoma and has provided remarkable outcomes for what was previously among most treatment refractory cancers. Immune checkpoint inhibitors play a key role, particularly when no targetable mutations are available. Harnessing the immune system against cancers, which is mediated by cytotoxic lymphocytes and the adaptive immune system, changed the landscape of melanoma therapy. The standard of care in the current era includes immune-modulating modalities such as PD-1 inhibitors (nivolumab and pembrolizumab) and CTLA-4 antibody inhibitors (ipilimumab). Clinical trials investigating these drugs have resulted in unprecedented outcomes in both metastatic and stage III melanomas with improvements in overall and PFS.

The landmark trial in 2010 by Hodi and colleagues[20] changed the way the scientific community approaches melanoma. This phase III study explored the CTLA-4 inhibitor ipilimumab in subjects with metastatic melanoma and found a 10-month improvement in OS, which was monumental compared with the disappointing outcomes seen in prior IL-2 therapies and chemotherapy. The 1-year and 2-year survival rates were 46% and 24%, respectively, compared with 25% and 14%, respectively, in the control group. Immediately after publication of this trial, ipilimumab was approved for the treatment of advanced melanoma.

PD-1 inhibitors have proven to be the most effective immunotherapies in melanoma, especially when combined with the CTLA-4 inhibitor ipilimumab. One of the earliest clinical trials exploring these PD-1 targeted antibodies was with nivolumab in the

CheckMate 066 trial. In this trial, 210 subjects with metastatic or unresectable melanoma had a 1-year survival rate of 72.9%, and median PFS was 5.1 months (median OS was not reached).[21] The Keynote-006 trial investigated pembrolizumab at a dosing of every 2 or 3 weeks versus ipilimumab every 3 weeks, and demonstrated a 1-year survival rate of 74.1%, 68.4%, and 58.2%, respectively.[22] Updated long-term analysis of this trial showed durable response to treatment with 91% of subjects who did not progress after 2 years. These trials demonstrated that both nivolumab and pembrolizumab have more favorable safety profiles compared with ipilimumab. Such extraordinary outcomes from PD-1 inhibitors have made these drugs the standard of care for subjects with metastatic or unresectable melanomas.

Furthermore, combination therapy with ipilimumab and PD-1 inhibitors have demonstrated a higher antitumor effect and increased inflammatory cell infiltration compared with ipilimumab alone. Dual blockade with nivolumab plus ipilimumab was first studied in the phase I dose-escalation study, CA209-004, by Wolchok and colleagues.[23] This study was later evaluated in a phase II (CheckMate 069) and phase III (CheckMate 067) clinical trials.[24,25] The objective response rate with combination therapy in the CA209-004 was 40%, which was higher than demonstrated with ipilimumab monotherapy (11%) or nivolumab monotherapy (28%). Updated 3-year analysis of the CA209-004 by Callahan and colleagues[26] in 2018, showed that combination therapy with nivolumab and ipilimumab in subjects with advanced unresectable melanoma had a 3-year OS rate of 63% with median OS not yet reached. The objective response rate was 42% in 3 years with median duration of response 22.3 months. Incidence of grade 3 and 4 toxicities occurred in 59% of subjects over the 3 years.

The phase III clinical trial (CheckMate 067) in 2015 by Larkin and colleagues[27] explored combination treatment with nivolumab and ipilimumab versus nivolumab alone versus ipilimumab alone in untreated unresectable stage III or stage IV subjects. The investigators found that PFS was 11.5 months in the nivolumab-ipilimumab group, but 14 months in subjects with PD-L1 (+) subjects and 11.2 months in PD-L1 (−) subjects. The nivolumab monotherapy cohort had a PFS of 6.9 months overall, with 14 months in the PD-L1 (+) group and 5.3 months in the PD-L1 (−) group. Ipilimumab monotherapy demonstrated a PFS of 2.9 months in the PD-L1 (+) group. In summary, in PD-L1 (+) subjects, combination nivolumab-ipilimumab was essentially equivalent to nivolumab alone but at the price of higher toxicity with the combination. In PD-L1 (−) tumors, nivolumab was superior. Between the 2 monotherapies, nivolumab was superior to ipilimumab. This confirmed the clinical benefit of combination therapy in the treatment of advanced melanomas.

A phase III study in 2015 evaluated immunotherapy in the adjuvant setting and showed that ipilimumab alone improved recurrence-free survival (RFS) by 10 months versus placebo in resected stage III melanomas.[28] Then, in 2017, Weber and colleagues[29] compared nivolumab to ipilimumab in this population and found that nivolumab had a significantly higher 12-month RFS of 70.5%, whereas ipilimumab had a 12-month RFS of 60.8%. In 2018, the PD-1 inhibitor, pembrolizumab, was studied against placebo in subjects with stage III resected melanoma and was found to have a significantly improved 12-month RFS rate of 75.4% with pembrolizumab compared with 61% with placebo.[30–44] The impressive responses seen in these trials led to the approval of PD-1 inhibitors as adjuvant treatment of melanoma.

GENETIC TESTING

A wide array of genetic and genomic aberrations has been identified in melanoma, most commonly *BRAF*, *NRAS*, and *KIT* mutations. Although many are point mutations, various types of genomic abnormalities exist, contributing to the vast heterogenicity of tumor cells. Identifying specific mutations is key to appropriate and effective targeted treatment, and is the backbone behind the concept and value of precision medicine. Traditionally, genetic testing techniques for identifying these aberrations included direct sequencing of DNA, which recognizes point mutations within a given portion of DNA. The single nucleotide extension assay is another molecular study that identifies known point mutations within a specific genetic region of interest; however, this technique will only detect mutations within the genetic region studied. Fluorescence in situ hybridization (FISH) detects greater areas of genomic aberrations, identifying larger gene amplifications, rearrangements, and deletions. There are a multitude of other genomic testing techniques that drive understanding of the genetic signature; however, none stand up to the merit of information made possible by massive parallel sequencing.

Massive parallel sequencing (ie, NGS) transcends the value over traditional molecular testing techniques. It provides simultaneous sequencing of entire exomes and genomes of tumor specimens, thus identifying essentially any subset of genetic and genomic aberration within the cancer cell. As expected, simultaneous sequencing of entire genetic material generates large amounts of data that are, in turn, analyzed and interpreted into the appropriate clinical application. This sophisticated process continues to evolve as research ensues within multiple research laboratories.

The most widely used and researched genomic profiling laboratories include Foundation One Medicine testing and Caris Life Sciences. They use several platforms of molecular and genetic testing for NGS. Analysis is usually performed on frozen tissue sections or blood-based samples. Dynamic light scattering, flow cytometry, fragment analysis, immunohistochemistry, and FISH are available in addition to NGS. In addition to these well-established syndicates, many academic institutions perform their own NGS testing with generalized panels with actionable mutations across all cancer types, whereas some use individualized panels. Exploratory data are often collected based on the institution's modified testing panel, which can be further used in research and institutional clinical trials.

NGS has revolutionized precision medicine and has led to the application of more effective therapies against several different types of cancer. It has helped to construct a comprehensive understanding of the genetic signatures of tumor cells, allowing for targeted treatment and better outcomes. In the study of melanoma, NGS identifies known genomic changes and somatic mutations, such as *BRAF*, *NRAS*, and *KIT* mutations. NGS also prompts the discovery of new genomic aberrations, which continue to be studied and refined as the vast library of data evolves.

Gene Expression Profiling

Another area in which genetic testing is starting to play a bigger role in the care of patients with melanoma is in gene expression profile (GEP) testing, which can provide essential prognostic information for patients with melanoma. The commonly used gene expression profile tests provided by Castle Biosciences stratify samples of both cutaneous and uveal melanomas into high and low risk of recurrence, metastasis, and survival based on the specific gene profile of that individual's melanoma. Although the American Joint Committee on Cancer (AJCC) staging allows for categorization of melanoma into distinct groups based on clinical and pathologic data that predict prognosis, the addition of personalized testing can enhance the accuracy of prognostication. Such results may lead to more informed and effective treatment plans.

The heterogeneity that characterizes the disease progression of melanoma has driven research aimed at identifying those patients with the highest risk of recurrence, metastasis, and mortality. The genetic mutations responsible for conferring malignant potential in melanoma have been investigated for nearly 2 decades as part of this search. Early studies determined that there are reproducible subsets of cutaneous melanoma based on certain genetic profiles.[1] Similarly, distinct classes of uveal melanoma based on gene expression profiles were also identified.[2] Subsets of cutaneous melanomas that included samples with high metastatic potential were further examined, highlighting genes and expressed sequence tags thought to play a role in disease progression and metastasis.[3-9] A comparative, retrospective analysis with samples of primary cutaneous melanoma and their respective metastasis added to the growing knowledge of metastatic pathways for cutaneous melanoma. Additionally, immunohistochemical markers associated with distant metastasis-free survival and OS were identified.[10]

The results from this research led to the development of GEP assays for both uveal and cutaneous melanoma used in clinical practice today. Difficulties in classification and prognostication of uveal melanoma led to rapid adoption of gene profiling. Early testing of a 3-gene signature showed superior prediction of metastatic death when compared with clinical and pathologic prognostic factors such as tumor thickness and presence of invasion, as well as chromosomal aberrations.[2] Additional studies supported these findings[11] and led to the development of a 15-gene GEP assay validated through a prospective multicenter study.[12,13] The studies illustrated a high technical success rate with 97% of cases classified and accurate prognostication of metastasis that outperformed any other prognostic factor (**Fig. 1**). Furthermore, the GEP assay demonstrated net reclassification improvements of 0.43 ($P = .001$) and 0.38 ($P = .004$) over the tumor-node-metastasis (TNM) classification and chromosome 3 status, respectively.

Although TNM staging for cutaneous melanoma provides critical prognostic information to patients and providers, there remains significant variability in the development of disease progression within the different stages.[14] In an effort to address this variability and identify patients at risk of metastases despite reassuring AJCC staging, a 31-gene signature was developed using published genomic anlyses.[15] Archived melanoma samples were classified into 2 groups, with class 1 and class 2 tumors indicating a low and high risk of metastasis, respectively. In a validation set of 104 cases of cutaneous melanoma, the negative predictive value (NPV) and positive predictive value (PPV) were found to be 93% and 72%, respectively. When including only stage I and stage II melanomas, as defined by the AJCC staging system, the NPV and PPV were 94% and 67%, respectively. The GEP assay was found to be an independent predictor of metastatic risk with a hazard ratio of 9.55 ($P = .002$). This compared favorably with the hazard ratio of 5.4 ($P = .002$) for AJCC staging. These findings were supported in follow-up prospective[16,17] and retrospecitve[18,19] trials in which the prognostic accuracy of the 31-gene GEP assay was evaluated. The trials have shown the ability of the assay to accurately risk-stratify patients independent of lymph node status. In a study by Gerami and colleagues[16] with subjects with a class 2 GEP signature, there was no statistical difference in DFS or OS for subjects with positive sentinel lymph nodes and those with negative sentinel lymph nodes (**Fig. 2**). Gene profiling may in fact replace sentinel lymph node status in some cases. A recent study by Vetto and colleagues[20] evaluated the ability of the 31-gene GEP assay to predict lymph node positivity. In subjects with T1-T2 tumors and low-risk gene profiles; that is, class 1, the rates of sentinel lymph node positivity in those aged greater than or equal to 65 years, 55 to 64 years, and less than 55 years were found to be 1.6%,

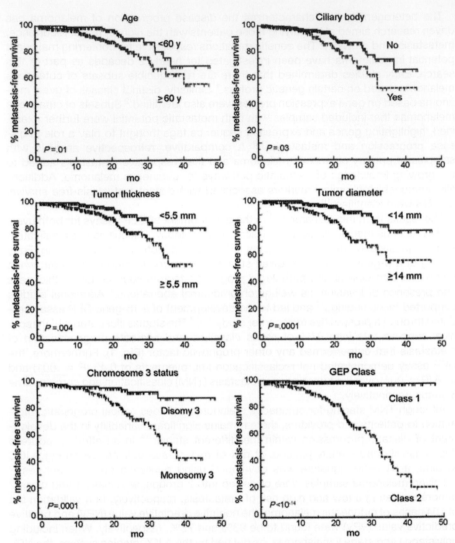

Fig. 1. Comparison of GEP classification with other prognostic factors. Kaplan-Meier plots for the indicated prognostic factors. *P* values were determined by the log-rank method. Age indicates patient's age at the time of the primary tumor diagnosis. Threshold values for dichotomizing continuous variables (tumor thickness and diameter) were determined by receiver operating characteristic analysis. (*From* B. R. Gastman, P. Gerami, S. J. Kurley, et al., Identification of patients at risk of metastasis using a prognostic 31-gene expression profile in subpopulations of melanoma patients with favorable outcomes by standard cirteria. Journal of the American Academy of Dermatology. 2019;1:80:149–157; with permission.)

4.9%, and 7.6%, respectively. These findings raise the question of whether sentinel lymph node biopsy can be avoided in certain patient populations with low-risk melanomas by GEP assay. The numbers of subjects involved in these studies are still low and require further validation.

In terms of prognostic information, GEP for cutaneous melanoma theoretically yields the most benefit for those with low AJCC stages but high metastatic potential.

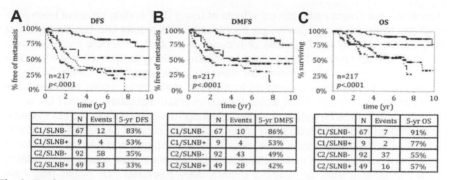

Fig. 2. Kaplan-Meier estimates of DFS (*A*), distant metastasis-free survival (DMFS) (*B*), and OS (*C*) in a cohort of 217 cutaneous melanoma cases with outcomes predicted by sentinel lymph node biopsy (SLNB) procedure in combination with GEP testing. Four subgroups of patients are described and shown after assignment of SLNB and GEP prognostic prediction. (*From* P. Gerami, R. W. Cook, M. C. Russell, et al. Gene expression profiling for molecular staging of cutaneous melanoma in patients undergoing sentinel lymph node biopsy. Journal of the American Academy of Dermatology. 2015; 5:72; 780–785; with permission.)

The hope is that by providing personalized evaluation of each melanoma case, clinicians can offer more appropriate treatment plans and follow-up to their patients. In the case of a patient with a stage I or IIA melanoma, a class 2 assignment may provide more realistic prognostic information. National Comprehensive Cancer Network (NCCN) guidelines do not recommend routine imaging as part of follow-up to screen for recurrence or metastasis in stage I or IIA patients, with no evidence of disease after wide local excision and do not recommend the use of GEP testing to inform follow-up screening.[45] It is hypothesized that the addition of class 2 prognostication may influence clinicians to obtain surveillance imaging and evaluate such a patient more regularly, outside of current NCCN algorithms. Additionally, such information may lead to recommendations for inclusion in clinical trials or administration of newer therapies that would not have been previously offered and which have shown improved survival for patients with more advanced disease.

The potential impact of GEP testing can be perceived when assessing outcomes in stage I or IIA patients specifically. In a study evaluating the development of a cutaneous melanoma GEP test, retrospective analysis of the test's predictive value in stage I and II patients was carried out.[46–51] Follow-up was at least 5 years or until a metastatic event. Out of 119 cases of stage I melanoma, 9 cases were found to have documented metastases. Of these 9 cases, 5 (56%) were accurately predicted to have a poor outcome based on being class 2 on GEP testing. Conversely, 5% of stage I patients without a metastatic event were inaccurately over-staged by the GEP assay and assigned to class 2. As the AJCC stage increased, the sensitivity of the GEP test increased but the specificity decreased. For patients with stage IIA (*n* = 45), IIB (*n* = 42), and IIC (*n* = 14) melanomas, 90% (19/21), 96% (27/28), and 100% (11/11), respectively, with metastatic events were appropriately assigned to the class 2 group. At the same time, the number of cases assigned class 2 in which there was no metastatic event by 5 years of follow-up steadily increased across stage II categories; 33% (8/24) of stage IIA, 57% (8/14) of stage IIB, and 67% (2/3) of stage IIC melanomas without metastases were class 2 on GEP testing. Importantly, the staging was not based on the most recent eighth edition of the AJCC system, but the differences between the seventh and eighth editions would not have affected stage II subjects.

Currently, the downstream clinical effects of using GEP testing have not been evaluated and there are no guidelines on how to translate results into decision-making. Thus, looking at the small sample previously described, providers must ask how GEP testing would have affected clinical decision-making for the 164 stage I and IIA patients. Out of those 164 patients, 38 were classified as class 2. Of the 24 stage I and IIA class 2 patients who went on to develop metastasis, would any have been offered additional therapies that would have prevented metastatic events? Or, would the metastatic events be detected earlier, allowing for expedient initiation of systemic therapy? Most importantly, do these changes lead to survival benefit? It is critical to also ask what the effect would have been for the 14 stage I and IIA class 2 patients who did not go on to have metastatic events. Would they have been inappropriately enrolled in clinical trials or received unnecessary therapies? Or would they have only received more regular follow-up and imaging? These are all questions that have yet to be answered.

SUMMARY

Precision medicine has transformed the treatment of melanoma and has provided more meaningful outcomes in a previously treatment-resistant cancer. It has driven changes in molecular testing strategies and clinical trial design, making targeted genetic aberrations the director of therapy for several cancers, notably in melanoma. GEP is helping to identify lower stage patients who may have a higher risk for metastases that may benefit from enhanced surveillance or even treatment. Targeted treatments specific for *BRAF*, *NRAS*, and *KIT* mutations, as well as the use of immunotherapies, have resulted in superior outcomes and survival in both advanced and adjuvant settings. Both monotherapies and combination therapies targeting these mutations have become the standard of care in melanoma, leaving chemotherapy and IL-2 therapy as third-line or greater treatment options when resistance to targeted therapies develops. Further investigations into a multitude of targeted combination therapies may represent opportunities to expand treatment options for patients with melanoma. In conclusion, precision medicine has brought about a new era in the treatment melanoma that continues to improve and evolve each year.

REFERENCES

1. Carvajal RD. Targeting KIT for treatment of advanced melanoma. The Melanoma Letter Winter 2011;29(3).
2. Johnson DB, Flaherty KT, Weber JS, et al. Combined BRAF (Dabrafenib) and MEK Inhibition (Trametinib) in patients with *BRAF*^{V600}-mutant melanoma experiencing progression with single-agent BRAF inhibitor. J Clin Oncol 2014;32(33): 3697–704.
3. Maio M, Lewis K, Demidov L, et al. Adjuvant vemurafenib in resected, BRAF V600 mutation-positive melanoma (BRIM8): a randomised, double-blind, placebo-controlled, multicentre, phase 3 trial. Lancet Oncol 2018;19(4):510–20.
4. Long GV, Hauschild A, Santinami M, et al. Adjuvant dabrafenib plus trametinib in Stage III *BRAF*-mutated melanoma. N Engl J Med 2017;377(19):1813–23.
5. Robert C, Karaszewska B, Schachter J, et al. Improved overall survival in melanoma with combined dabrafenib and trametinib. N Engl J Med 2015;372(1):30–9.
6. Larkin J, Ascierto PA, Dréno B, et al. Combined vemurafenib and cobimetinib in *BRAF*-mutated melanoma. N Engl J Med 2014;371(20):1867–76.
7. Chapman PB, Hauschild A, Robert C, et al. Improved survival with vemurafenib in melanoma with BRAF V600E mutation. N Engl J Med 2011;364(26):2507–16.

8. Chapman PB, Robert C, Larkin J, et al. Vemurafenib in patients with BRAFV600 mutation-positive metastatic melanoma: final overall survival results of the randomized BRIM-3 study. Ann Oncol 2017;28(10):2581–7.

9. Ascierto PA, Minor D, Ribas A, et al. Phase II trial (BREAK-2) of the BRAF inhibitor dabrafenib (GSK2118436) in patients with metastatic melanoma. J Clin Oncol 2013;31(26):3205–11.

10. Hauschild A, Grob JJ, Demidov LV, et al. Phase III, randomized, open-label, multicenter trial (BREAK-3) comparing the BRAF kinase inhibitor dabrafenib (GSK2118436) with dacarbazine (DTIC) in patients with BRAF ^{V600E} -mutated melanoma. J Clin Oncol 2012;30(18):LBA8500.

11. Chapman PB, Ascierto PA, Schadendorf D, et al. "Updated 5-y landmark analyses of phase 2 (BREAK-2) and phase 3 (BREAK-3) studies evaluating dabrafenib monotherapy in patients with BRAF V600–mutant melanoma. J Clin Oncol 2017;35(15_suppl):9526.

12. Dummer R, Ascierto PA, Gogas HJ, et al. Encorafenib plus binimetinib versus vemurafenib or encorafenib in patients with BRAF -mutant melanoma (COLUMBUS): a multicentre, open-label, randomised phase 3 trial. Lancet Oncol 2018; 19(5):603–15.

13. Johnson DB, Lovly CM, Flavin M, et al. Impact of NRAS mutations for patients with advanced melanoma treated with immune therapies. Cancer Immunol Res 2015; 3(3):288–95.

14. Muñoz-Couselo E, Zamora Adelantado E, Ortiz Vélez C, et al. NRAS-mutant melanoma: current challenges and future prospect. Onco Targets Ther 2017;10: 3941–7.

15. Kirkwood JM, Bastholt L, Robert C, et al. Phase II, open-label, randomized trial of the MEK1/2 inhibitor selumetinib as monotherapy versus temozolomide in patients with advanced melanoma. Clin Cancer Res 2012;18(2):555–67.

16. Robert C, Dummer R, Gutzmer R, et al. Selumetinib plus dacarbazine versus placebo plus dacarbazine as first-line treatment for BRAF-mutant metastatic melanoma: a phase 2 double-blind randomised study. Lancet Oncol 2013;14(8): 733–40.

17. Dummer R, Schadendorf D, Ascierto PA, et al. Binimetinib versus dacarbazine in patients with advanced NRAS -mutant melanoma (NEMO): a multicentre, open-label, randomised, phase 3 trial. Lancet Oncol 2017;18(4):435–45.

18. Guo J, Si L, Kong Y, et al. Phase II, open-label, single-arm trial of imatinib mesylate in patients with metastatic melanoma harboring c-Kit mutation or amplification. J Clin Oncol 2011;29(21):2904–9.

19. Carvajal RD. KIT as a therapeutic target in metastatic melanoma. JAMA 2011; 305(22):2327.

20. Hodi FS, O'Day SJ, McDermott DF, et al. Improved survival with ipilimumab in patients with metastatic melanoma. N Engl J Med 2010;363(8):711–23.

21. Robert C, Long GV, Brady B, et al. Nivolumab in previously untreated melanoma without BRAF mutation. N Engl J Med 2015;372(4):320–30.

22. Robert C, Schachter J, Long GV, et al. Pembrolizumab versus ipilimumab in advanced melanoma. N Engl J Med 2015;372(26):2521–32.

23. Wolchok JD, Kluger H, Callahan MK, et al. Nivolumab plus ipilimumab in advanced melanoma. N Engl J Med 2013;369(2):122–33.

24. Postow MA, Chesney J, Pavlick AC, et al. Nivolumab and Ipilimumab versus Ipilimumab in Untreated Melanoma. N Engl J Med 2015;372(21):2006–17.

25. Hodi FS, Chesney J, Pavlick AC, et al. Combined nivolumab and ipilimumab versus ipilimumab alone in patients with advanced melanoma: 2-year overall

survival outcomes in a multicentre, randomised, controlled, phase 2 trial. Lancet Oncol 2016;17(11):1558–68.

26. Callahan MK, Kluger H, Postow MA, et al. Nivolumab plus ipilimumab in patients with advanced melanoma: updated survival, response, and safety data in a phase I dose-escalation study. J Clin Oncol 2018;36(4):391–8.

27. Larkin J, Chiarion-Sileni V, Gonzalez R, et al. Combined nivolumab and ipilimumab or monotherapy in untreated melanoma. N Engl J Med 2015;373(1):23–34.

28. Eggermont AMM, Chiarion-Sileni V, Grob J-J, et al. Adjuvant ipilimumab versus placebo after complete resection of high-risk stage III melanoma (EORTC 18071): a randomised, double-blind, phase 3 trial. Lancet Oncol 2015;16(5): 522–30.

29. Weber J, Mandala M, Del Vecchio M, et al. Adjuvant nivolumab versus ipilimumab in resected stage III or IV melanoma. N Engl J Med 2017;377(19):1824–35.

30. Eggermont AMM, Blank CU, Mandala M, et al. Adjuvant pembrolizumab versus placebo in resected stage III melanoma. N Engl J Med 2018;378(19):1789–801.

31. Bittner M, Meltzer P, Chen Y, et al. Molecular classification of cutaneous malignant melanoma by gene expression profiling. Nature 2000;406:536–40.

32. Onken MD, Worley LA, Ehlers JP, et al. Gene expression profiling in uveal melanoma reveals two molecular classes and predicts metastatic death. Cancer Res 2004;64:7205–9.

33. Clark EA, Golub TR, Lander ES, et al. Genomic analysis of metastasis reveals an essential role for RhoC. Nature 2000;406:532–5.

34. Weeraratna AT, Jiang Y, Hostetter G, et al. Wnt5a signaling directly affects cell motility and invasion of metastatic melanoma. Cancer Cell 2002;1:279–88.

35. Haqq C, Nosrati M, Sudilovsky D, et al. The gene expression signatures of melanoma progression. Proc Natl Acad Sci U S A 2005;102:6092–7.

36. Smith AP, Hoek K, Becker D. Whole-genome expression profiling of the melanoma progression pathway reveals marked molecular differences between nevi/melanoma in situ and advanced-stage melanomas. Cancer Biol Ther 2005;4:1018–29.

37. Jaeger J, Koczan D, Thiesen H-J, et al. Gene expression signatures for tumor progression, tumor subtype, and tumor thickness in laser-microdissected melanoma tissues. Clin Cancer Res 2007;13:806–15.

38. Scatolini M, Grand MM, Grosso E, et al. Altered molecular pathways in melanocytic lesions. Int J Cancer 2010;126:1869–81.

39. Mauerer A, Roesch A, Hafner C, et al. Identification of new genes associated with melanoma. Exp Dermatol 2011;20:502–7.

40. Winnepenninckx V, Lazar V, Michiels S, et al. Gene expression profiling of primary cutaneous melanoma and clinical outcome. J Natl Cancer Inst 2006. https://doi.org/10.1093/jnci/djj103.

41. Petrausch U, Martus P, Tö Nnies H, et al. Significance of gene expression analysis in uveal melanoma in comparison to standard risk factors for risk assessment of subsequent metastases. Eye 2008;22:997–1007.

42. Onken MD, Worley LA, Tuscan MD, et al. An accurate, clinically feasible multigene expression assay for predicting metastasis in uveal melanoma. J Mol Diagn 2010;12:461–8.

43. Onken MD, Worley LA, Char DH, et al. Collaborative ocular oncology group report number 1: prospective validation of a multi-gene prognostic assay in uveal melanoma. Ophthalmology 2012. https://doi.org/10.1016/j.ophtha.2012.02.017.

44. Svedman FC, Pillas D, Taylor A, et al. Stage-specific survival and recurrence in patients with cutaneous malignant melanoma in Europe - a systematic review of the literature. Clin Epidemiol 2016;8:109–22.

45. NCCN clinical practice guidelines in oncology (NCCN Guidelines®) for cutaneous melanoma V.2.2019. National Comprehensive Cancer Network, Inc.; 2019. Accessed March 12, 2019.

46. Gerami P, Cook RW, Wilkinson J, et al. Development of a prognostic genetic signature to predict the metastatic risk associated with cutaneous melanoma. Clin Cancer Res 2015. https://doi.org/10.1158/1078-0432.CCR-13-3316.

47. Gerami P, Cook RW, Russell MC, et al. Gene expression profiling for molecular staging of cutaneous melanoma in patients undergoing sentinel lymph node biopsy. J Am Acad Dermatol 2015. https://doi.org/10.1016/j.jaad.2015.01.009.

48. Hsueh EC, DeBloom JR, Lee J, et al. Interim analysis of survival in a prospective, multi-center registry cohort of cutaneous melanoma tested with a prognostic 31-gene expression profile test. J Hematol Oncol 2017;10:152.

49. Zager JS, Gastman BR, Leachman S, et al. Performance of a prognostic 31-gene expression profile in an independent cohort of 523 cutaneous melanoma patients. BMC Cancer 2018;18:130.

50. Gastman BR, Zager JS, Messina JL, et al. Performance of a 31-gene expression profile test in cutaneous melanomas of the head and neck. Head Neck 2019;41: 871–9.

51. Vetto JT, Hsueh EC, Gastman BR, et al. Guidance of sentinel lymph node biopsy decisions in patients with T1–T2 melanoma using gene expression profiling. Future Oncol 2019;15:1207–17.

Precision Medicine in Lung Cancer Treatment

Dhaval R. Shah, MBBS, MD[a], Gregory A. Masters, MD[a,b],*

KEYWORDS

- Lung cancer • Immunotherapy • Targeted therapy • Molecular testing
- Clinical trials

KEY POINTS

- Lung cancer remains leading cause of cancer death in men and women in the United States and more than 80% of these patients have non-small cell lung cancer.
- Platinum-based doublet chemotherapy has been the standard treatment for patients with stage IV non-small cell lung cancer.
- Over the past 5 years, immunotherapy has rapidly changed management of stage IV lung cancer and is now being used as frontline treatment option with or without chemotherapy.
- It is being used as consolidation treatment in management of patients with stage III non-small cell lung cancer after completion of chemotherapy and radiation.
- Immunotherapy is approved for use in patients with extensive stage small cell lung cancer.

INTRODUCTION

Lung cancer is the second most common cancer in men and women, and according to American Cancer Society, approximately 228,150 new cases of lung cancer will be diagnosed in 2019 in the United States. An estimated 142,670 deaths will be attributed to lung cancer in 2019. There are 3 main types of lung cancer, non-small cell lung cancer (NSCLC), small cell lung cancer (SCLC), and lung carcinoid tumor. NSCLC accounts for approximately 85% of new cases, SCLC accounts for approximately 10% to 15% of cases, and carcinoid tumors are less than 5% of new cases.[1] Unfortunately, more than 50% of cases are diagnosed in the advanced stage or stage IV.

Traditionally, the treatment for advanced NSCLC has been chemotherapy. Updated guidelines from the American Society of Clinical Oncology support these recommendations.[2] However, in the past decade, tremendous advances have been made in understanding the biology and genetic drivers in NSCLC. As a result, many targeted and

---

Disclosure Statement: None.
[a] Helen F. Graham Cancer Center and Research Institute, 4701 Ogletown-Stanton Road, Newark, DE 19713, USA; [b] Thomas Jefferson University Medical School, Philadelphia, PA, USA
* Corresponding author. Helen F. Graham Cancer Center and Research Institute, 4701 Ogletown-Stanton Road, Newark, DE 19713.
E-mail address: Gregory.Masters@usoncology.com

Surg Oncol Clin N Am 29 (2020) 15–21
https://doi.org/10.1016/j.soc.2019.08.002
1055-3207/20/© 2019 Elsevier Inc. All rights reserved.

immunotherapy drugs are now being used in the management of advanced NSCLC. These drugs are also being incorporated in early stage lung cancer, with the hope of improving outcomes and cure rates in patients with stages I to III lung cancer.

ADVANCED OR STAGE IV NON-SMALL CELL LUNG CANCER

NSCLC is divided into different histologic subtypes, which include adenocarcinoma, large cell carcinoma, and squamous cell carcinoma. Traditionally, platinum-based doublet chemotherapy has been the standard of care in advanced NSCLC. However, Scagliotti and colleagues[3] established the importance of histology in the treatment of advanced NSCLC, showing the advantage of pemetrexed in combination with a platinum agent as first-line treatment in nonsquamous NSCLC histologic subtype. Taxane with a platinum agent is the preferred chemotherapy combination for squamous histology.

Similarly, molecular characterization of NSCLC has become increasingly important as a predictive and prognostic marker to guide therapy. In 2004, an epidermal growth factor receptor (EGFR) mutation was the first molecular target identified in a subgroup of patients with NSCLC, and was associated with significant responses to oral tyrosine kinase inhibitor (TKI) geftinib.[4] Two other TKIs, erlotinib and afatinib, were also shown to be very effective in this subgroup of patients. EGFR TKIs are superior and improve survival as compared with chemotherapy in patients with stage IV NSCLC with certain EGFR mutations. Almost all of these patients will eventually progress and about one-half of them will have a secondary T790M mutation. Osimertinib has been shown to be very effective in T790M mutation, and is the second-line treatment of choice in these patients.[5] In 2018, Soria and colleagues[6] reported superior outcomes with osimertinib compared with first-generation TKIs (erlotinib and geftinib) as first-line treatment for untreated patients with EGFR mutation. Based on this, the US Food and Drug Administration has approved osimertinib for frontline use in EGFR mutant advanced NSCLC.

Similar to the EGFR mutation, EML4-ALK fusion was found to be another targetable gene alteration in small subgroup of patients with advanced nonsquamous NSCLC. EML4-ALK fusion oncogene leads to aberrant activation of EML4-ALK protein and it was first reported in 2007. Crizotinib was the first TKI shown to be effective in this subgroup of patients in 2010.[7] It was then found to be superior to standard chemotherapy in previously untreated ALK-positive NSCLC.[8] Other active TKI drugs include alectinib, certinib, and brigatinib. The ALEX study compared alectinib with crizotinib in untreated patients with EML4-ALK fusion, and showed significant improvement in survival with alectinib.[9] Thus, alectinib is now considered as the preferred first-line treatment option in treatment-naïve patients with this fusion. In patients, who are initially treated with crizotinib, treatment can be changed to second-generation TKIs, such as certinib or brigatinib.

ROS-1 rearrangement and BRAF mutation are other targetable mutations in advanced NSCLC. Crizotinib and certinib are effective in treatment of ROS-1 mutated NSCLC. The combination of dabrafenib and trametinib is considered a first-line or second-line treatment option in patients with advanced NSCLC with BRAF V600E mutation. More recently, larotrectinib has been shown to be a treatment option in patients with NTRK gene fusion,[10] and can be used in patients with lung cancer with this gene fusion.

Given these rapid advancements in the treatment of advanced NSCLC, molecular testing has become very important to choose the correct treatment approach. This molecular testing can be done by different methods, such as hotspot testing for specific genes, or more comprehensive gene sequencing of the tumors. The College of

American Pathologists and the International Association for the Study of Lung Cancer recommend upfront testing for EGFR, ALK, and ROS-1 mutations in all patients with advanced nonsquamous NSCLC.[11] Routine testing for BRAF, RET, HER2, KRAS, and MET genes is not considered as a standard, but can be done as part of a gene sequencing panel. The College of American Pathologists/International Association for the Study of Lung Cancer and the American Society of Clinical Oncology guidelines both recommend use of multiplex gene panels (where available) for identifying mutations beyond EGFR, ALK, ROS-1, and BRAF.

Many patients with advanced NSCLC do not have enough biopsy tissue to run all the hotspot or gene sequencing studies listed. Therefore, more recently liquid biopsy or peripheral blood-based genetic testing has been shown to be effective in detection of these gene alterations.[12] The principle behind liquid biopsy is detection of cell free circulating DNA, which is often present in the blood of patients with cancer. This method has most commonly been studied for EGFR mutation, and the US Food and Drug Administration has approved 2 tests for this use. Data are rapidly emerging regarding use of liquid biopsy in testing for other molecular targets.

Despite the advancements in the identification of these molecular targets, the majority of patients with advanced NSCLC do not harbor these mutations. Frontline platinum-based doublet chemotherapy used to be the standard of care for these patients. Immunotherapeutic agents have rapidly changed this standard over the past 5 years. These immune checkpoint inhibitors alter the tumor microenvironment and remove the blockade of the immune system evasion by cancer cells.

One of the mechanisms of the human immune system to eliminate malignant cells is through formation of cancer-specific T cells. Antigen-presenting cells such as natural killer cells and macrophages penetrate the tumor microenvironment, and activate the T cells, which in turn destroy cancer cells. However, in cancer, 2 normal inhibitory pathways (CTLA-4 and programmed death 1 [PD-1] pathways) have been found to suppress this T-cell response. Ipilimumab, an anti–CTLA-4 monoclonal antibody, was the first immune checkpoint inhibitor developed in the treatment of cancer. However, CTLA-4 is an immunoglobulin, which is expressed on activated T cells in many normal and cancer cells, and therefore ipilimumab can be associated with significant inflammatory and autoimmune toxicities. PD-1 receptor pathway is the second mechanism that controls the T-cell immune response. PD-1 gets expressed on the surface of the T cells after persistent antigen exposure, and then interacts with its ligand PD-L1, which is expressed on both immune and cancer cells. This interaction causes inhibition of T-cell activation and response. PD-1 activation normally affects the effector T cells and cytotoxic lymphocytes, which are seen in the lymph node and tumor microenvironment. Inhibition of PD-1 and PD ligand 1 (PD-L1) pathway can therefore lead to prolonged antitumor response and many PD-1 and PD-L1 antibodies have been approved for clinical use.

PD-L1 expression has been found to correlate with response to immunotherapy drugs. In general, higher PD-L1 expression is associated with higher and long-term response.[13] Testing for PD-L1 expression is now standard in all newly diagnosed patients with advanced NSCLC. Tumor mutation burden is the number of mutations seen in the cancer cells' DNA. A higher tumor mutation burden is also associated with better response to immunotherapy. Similarly, microsatellite instability has been shown to be associated with good response to immunotherapy. Most commercial laboratories now report PD-L1 expression, tumor mutation burden, and microsatellite instability status as part of comprehensive gene sequencing report.

Initial studies evaluating immunotherapy drugs in lung cancer were done in the second line setting after progression on platinum doublet chemotherapy. The CheckMate

017 and CheckMate 057 trials showed statistically significant improvement in overall survival with nivolumab compared with docetaxel in squamous and nonsquamous NSCLC, respectively.[14,15] Overall survival was improved by approximately 3 months in both the trials. The KEYNOTE-010 trial showed significant improvement in overall survival with pembrolizumab compared with docetaxel in second line treatment for advanced NSCLC with at least 1% PD-L1 expression in the tumor cells.[16] Based on these trials, initial approval for both nivolumab and pembrolizumab was in the second line setting after progression on first line chemotherapy. Pembrolizumab was approved for patients with PD-L1 overexpression only.

Given the improvement in survival in the second-line setting, pembrolizumab was studied in combination with carboplatin and pemetrexed in first line setting in patients with nonsquamous NSCLC, with no driver mutations. This Keynote 189 trial also included maintenance treatment with pemetrexed and pembrolizumab.[17] Significant improvement in overall survival was noted with addition of pembrolizumab to chemotherapy, and is now considered as the standard of care for first-line treatment in nonsquamous advanced NSCLC, irrespective of the PD-L1 status. Pembrolizumab in combination with chemotherapy has also shown to improve survival in patients with metastatic squamous cell NSCLC regardless of PD-L1 expression and is standard of care as a first-line treatment option.[18] The Keynote-042 trial evaluated pembrolizumab alone as first-line therapy versus chemotherapy in stage IV NSCLC, and pembrolizumab was associated with a significant improvement in overall survival. Based on this trial, pembrolizumab alone is also a treatment option for patients with advanced NSCLC and PD-L1 expression or more than 1%. It seems to be most active in tumors with PD-L1 of 50% or greater.

Similarly, the IMpower 150 clinical trial evaluated atezolizumab, which is an anti–PD-L1 antibody, in combination with carboplatin, paclitaxel, and bevacizumab in metastatic nonsquamous NSCLC.[19] This combination also showed improved survival and is another front-line treatment option for patients with nonsquamous NSCLC. Thus, immunotherapy has rapidly changed the management of metastatic NSCLC over the past 5 years.

Despite this rapid progress in the management of NSCLC, most patients eventually have progression of disease; the median survival in these trials is generally 2 years or less. Several trials are ongoing looking at other molecular targets in lung cancer and other solid tumors. Two such large trials are the NCI-MATCH (Molecular Analysis for Therapy Choice) study and American Society of Clinical Oncology's Targeted Agent and Profiling Utilization Registry (TAPUR) study. Similarly the LUNG-MAP (SWOG S1400) study is a multidrug, targeted screening approach for patients with advanced NSCLC. The study matches patients to one of the multiple trial substudies, each testing a different drug based on molecular testing results. This study is a unique collaboration between the National Cancer Institute, academic institutions, and private industry.

MANAGEMENT OF STAGES I TO III NON-SMALL CELL LUNG CANCER

Surgery remains the standard of care of most patients with stage I and stage II NSCLC. However, many patients are not candidates for surgery because of their functional status, medical comorbidities or underlying lung disease. Stereotactic body radiation has rapidly evolved as a treatment option for them and has been shown to have durable disease and long-term control.[20]

In patients who undergo surgery, adjuvant chemotherapy is generally recommended in patients with tumors greater than 4 cm or those with positive lymph nodes.

The standard adjuvant chemotherapy is a cisplatin-based combination regimen. Given the success with targeted and immunotherapy in advanced disease, these treatments are now being studied in early stage lung cancer. The ALCHEMIST (Adjuvant Lung Cancer Enrichment Marker Identification and Sequencing Trials) trial is looking at use of EGFR or ALK inhibitors or nivolumab in the adjuvant setting for patients with resected early stage NSCLC. In this trial, patients with EGFR or ALK mutations are randomly assigned to targeted therapy or observation after resection and any adjuvant chemotherapy. Patients without these mutations are randomly assigned to receive nivolumab or observation after resection and adjuvant chemotherapy.

The Keynote-671 trial is evaluating the safety and efficacy of pembrolizumab in combination with platinum doublet chemotherapy in the neoadjuvant and adjuvant settings. In this trial, patients with resectable stage IIB or IIIA NSCLC will be randomized to neoadjuvant chemotherapy with or without pembrolizumab, followed by surgery and then adjuvant pembrolizumab or placebo. This study started in 2018, with anticipated completion in 2024.

The management of patients with stage III NSCLC generally involves a multidisciplinary approach, involving surgical, medical, and radiation oncology. Some patients with early stage IIIA NSCLC undergo surgery, followed by adjuvant chemotherapy with or without radiation. However, patients with unresectable stage IIIA and more advanced stage IIIB and IIIC lung cancers are generally treated with a combination of chemotherapy and radiation. Most of these patients ultimately have progression of disease. To improve outcomes in these patients, the PACIFIC trial looked at using an anti–PDL-1 antibody durvalumab as consolidation therapy in patients with unresectable stage III NSCLC who did not have progression of disease after 2 or more cycles of platinum-based chemoradiotherapy. The trial showed a progression-free survival of 16.8 months for patients who received durvalumab versus a progression-free survival of 5.6 months with placebo. The updated analysis of the trial published in 2018 also showed a significant improvement in overall survival, and consolidation durvalumab is now considered a standard of care after chemotherapy and radiation.[21] New clinical trials will investigate the integration of immunotherapy earlier in a combined modality approach.

MANAGEMENT OF SMALL CELL LUNG CANCER

SCLC is typically divided into limited stage and extensive stage. Limited stage SCLC is treated with a combination of chemotherapy and radiation. Generally, the chemotherapy regimen of choice in this situation is cisplatin and etoposide. However, in older patients, and in patients with renal dysfunction, often carboplatin is used instead of cisplatin.

The management of extensive stage SCLC generally involves combination chemotherapy. Carboplatin and etoposide have been the standard of care for many years. The IMpower133 trial showed improvement in survival with the addition of atezolizumab immunotherapy drug to carboplatin and etoposide. Atezolizumab was given in combination with chemotherapy for the first 4 cycles, and then given as maintenance treatment.[22] This is now a standard of care in the management of extensive stage SCLC.

A similar concept of maintenance treatment is being studied with use of rovalpituzumab tesirine (Rova-T). Rovalpituzumab tesirine is an antibody drug conjugate, which targets the delta-like protein 3 inhibitory notch receptor expressed in SCLC. Similar other concepts will be studied in the future to improve outcomes in patients with SCLC.

FUTURE

As we move on to the next generation of clinical trials, increasing flexibility will be required to keep up with the rapid advancements in testing and new knowledge. Despite the success seen with immunotherapy, only a small percentage of patients are seeing durable and long-term responses. We therefore need better biomarkers to predict and improve response to immunotherapy. Similarly, combination of antibody–drug conjugates with chemotherapy or immunotherapy will be important to study in the future. In addition, education of community and practicing oncologists will be critical to maximize the benefits to our patients.

SUMMARY

Over the past decade, tremendous progress has been made in understanding the molecular and biologic drivers of lung cancer. Testing for various biomarkers in lung cancer is improving our ability to understand the behavior of different cancers, so we can identify the optimal treatment strategy for each clinical subset of patients. This progress has helped us to deliver individualized precision therapy options for our patients with lung cancer. Ongoing clinical trials will help to improve our ability to offer our patients the most effective treatments to improve their survival and quality of life.

REFERENCES

1. American Cancer Society. Facts & figures 2019. Atlanta (GA): American Cancer Society; 2019.
2. Hanna N, Johnson D, Temin S, et al. Systemic therapy for stage IV non-small-cell lung cancer: American Society of Clinical Oncology clinical practice guideline update. J Clin Oncol 2017;35(30):3484–515.
3. Scagliotti GV, Parikh P, von Pawel J, et al. Phase III study comparing cisplatin plus gemcitabine with cisplatin plus pemetrexed in chemotherapy-naive patients with advanced-stage non-small-cell lung cancer. J Clin Oncol 2008;26:3543–51.
4. Lynch TJ, Bell DW, Sordella R, et al. Activating mutations in the epidermal growth factor receptor underlying responsiveness of non-small-cell lung cancer to gefitinib. N Engl J Med 2004;350(21):2129–39.
5. Goss G, Tsai CM, Shepherd FA, et al. Osimertinib for pretreated EGFR Thr790Met-positive advanced non-small-cell lung cancer (AURA2): a multicentre, open-label, single-arm, phase 2 study. Lancet Oncol 2016;17(12):1643–52.
6. Soria JC, Ohe Y, Vansteenkiste J, et al. Osimertinib in untreated EGFR-mutated advanced non-small-cell lung cancer. N Engl J Med 2018;378(2):113–25.
7. Kwak EL, Bang YJ, Cambridge DR, et al. Anaplastic lymphoma kinase inhibition in non-small-cell lung cancer. N Engl J Med 2010;363(18):1693–703.
8. Solomon BJ, Mok T, Kim DW, et al. First-line crizotinib versus chemotherapy in ALK-positive lung cancer. N Engl J Med 2014;371(23):2167–77.
9. Peters S, Camidge DR, Shaw AT, et al. Alectinib versus Crizotinib in untreated ALK-positive non-small-cell lung cancer. N Engl J Med 2017;377(9):829.
10. Hong DS, Bauer TM, Lee JJ, et al. Larotrectinib in adult patients with solid tumours: a multi-centre, open-label, phase I dose-escalation study. Ann Oncol 2019;30(2):325–31.
11. Lindeman NI, Cagle PT, Aisner DL, et al. Updated molecular testing guideline for the selection of lung cancer patients for treatment with targeted tyrosine kinase inhibitors: guideline from the College of American Pathologists, the International

Association for the Study of Lung Cancer, and the Association for Molecular Pathology. J Mol Diagn 2018;20(2):129–59.

12. Aggarwal C, Thompson JC, Black TA, et al. Clinical implications of plasma-based genotyping with the delivery of personalized therapy in metastatic non-small cell lung cancer. JAMA Oncol 2018. https://doi.org/10.1001/jamaoncol.2018.4305.

13. Herbst RS, Soria JC, Kowanetz M, et al. Predictive correlates of response to the anti-PD-L1 antibody MPDL3280A in cancer patients. Nature 2014;515(7528): 563–7.

14. Brahmer J, Reckamp KL, Baas P, et al. Nivolumab versus Docetaxel in advanced squamous-cell non-small-cell lung cancer. N Engl J Med 2015;373:123–35.

15. Borghaei H, Paz-Ares L, Horn L, et al. Nivolumab versus Docetaxel in advanced nonsquamous non-small-cell lung cancer. N Engl J Med 2015;373:1627–39.

16. Herbst RS, Baas P, Kim DW, et al. Pembrolizumab versus docetaxel for previously treated, PD-L1-positive, advanced non-small-cell lung cancer (KEYNOTE-010): a randomised controlled trial. Lancet 2016;387(10027):1540–50.

17. Gandhi L, Rodríguez-Abreu D, Gadgeel S, et al. Pembrolizumab plus chemotherapy in metastatic non-small-cell lung cancer. N Engl J Med 2018;378: 2078–92.

18. Paz-Ares L, Luft A, Vicente D, et al. Pembrolizumab plus chemotherapy for squamous non-small-cell lung cancer. N Engl J Med 2018;379:2040–51.

19. Socinski M, Jotte RM, Cappuzzo F, et al. Atezolizumab for first-line treatment of metastatic nonsquamous NSCLC. N Engl J Med 2018;378:2288–301.

20. Timmerman RD, Paulus R, Pass HI, et al. Stereotactic body radiation therapy for operable early-stage lung cancer: findings from the NRG oncology RTOG 0618 trial. JAMA Oncol 2018;4(9):1263–6.

21. Antonio SJ, Villegas A, Daniel D, et al. Overall survival with durvalumab after chemoradiotherapy in stage III NSCLC. N Engl J Med 2018;379:2342–50.

22. Horn L, Mansfield AS, Szczęsna A, et al. First-line atezolizumab plus chemotherapy in extensive-stage small-cell lung cancer. N Engl J Med 2018;379: 2220–9.

Precision Medicine in Colorectal Surgery

Sangeetha Prabhakaran, MD[a], Joseph Leong, BS[b], Nicholas J. Petrelli, MD[c,d], Vijay P. Khatri, MBChB, MBA[b,*]

KEYWORDS

• Precision medicine • Colorectal surgery • Predictive biomarkers

KEY POINTS

• There have been significant advances in the development of precision medicine for colorectal carcinoma, influencing areas of screening, treatment, and potentially prevention.

• Advances in molecular techniques have made it possible for better patient selection for therapies and it is important that mutational analysis be performed at the time of diagnosis to guide treatment.

• Future efforts should focus on validating these treatments in specific subgroups of colorectal tumors and on deeper understanding of the mechanisms of resistance to therapies.

• This will subsequently enable treatment optimization, promote efficacy, and reduce treatment costs and toxicities.

Despite significant improvements over the past decades, colorectal cancer (CRC) continues to be a leading cause of cancer-related death in the United States, with an estimated 51,020 deaths from CRC in the year 2019.[1] Selecting the appropriate treatment requires multidisciplinary team efforts that consider patients' characteristics, tumor genomics, and treatment goals.

PRECISION MEDICINE IN PREVENTION AND SCREENING

More than half (55%) of CRCs in the United States are attributable to potentially modifiable risk factors that include higher body mass index, sedentary lifestyle, smoking,

Disclosure: None.
[a] Division of Surgical Oncology, Department of Surgery, University of New Mexico, Albuquerque, NM, USA; [b] Department of Surgery, California Northstate University College of Medicine, Elk Grove, CA 95757, USA; [c] Department of Surgery, Helen F. Graham Cancer Center & Research Institute, Christiana Care Health System, Newark, DE, USA; [d] Department of Surgery, Thomas Jefferson University, Philadelphia, PA, USA
* Corresponding author. California Northstate University College of Medicine, Elk Grove, CA 95757.
E-mail address: vijay.khatri@cnsu.edu

alcohol consumption, consumption of red or processed meat, lower intake of calcium, fruits, vegetables and whole grain fiber.[1]

Non-modifiable risk factors include a personal or family history of CRC, adenomatous polyps, genetic conditions such as Lynch syndrome, a personal history of chronic inflammatory bowel disease and type-2 diabetes. Screening guidelines from the American Cancer Society recommend people with average risk for CRC begin screening at 45 years of age up to age 85 years, depending on health status and life expectancy. More individualized decision-making is recommended for ages 76 to 85 years based on patient preferences and prior screening history.[1]

Current screening guidelines for CRC stratify individuals into 4 risk groups primarily based on age and family history: high, moderate, average, and low. However, there remains intergroup heterogeneity based on genomic and environmental factors. A better understanding of molecular mechanisms that initiate cancer and drive progression has led to recent innovation in a molecular approach to precision prevention. Possible biomarkers to explore include metabolomic, proteomic, genomic, or epigenomic changes; and circulating cell free DNA; circulating tumor DNA (ctDNA); and circulating tumor cells. These are ideal as they provide a noninvasive method to detect disease. In particular, genomic characterization of CRC may allow for a more precise approach to screening.[2] The future of CRC screening will be risk-stratified algorithms that integrate genomic and lifestyle risk factors to create a more individualized risk profile with the goal to reduce overdiagnosis while maximizing detection of lesions with a high chance of progression to cancer.

Based on the Human Development Index, high-income countries (HICs) exhibit tumor types distinct from prevalence in low-income and middle-income counties; female breast, prostate, lung, and CRC are common is HICs. As developing countries undergo economic transition, so do the pattern of cancer types. Particularly for CRC, a principle challenge is engaging the community at risk and optimizing screening strategies. An emerging strategy to address the rising cancer burden has involved tumor-specific genomics, leading to targeted therapy and precision prevention. A molecular approach to early diagnosis and screening may be used to identify high-risk individuals providing risk-stratified algorithms for screening methods. For example, genome-wide association studies (GWASs) have already identified susceptibility loci for different tumor types, exemplified by colorectal and breast cancer.[3] Omic technology has provided the first integrated proteogenomic analysis, involving CRC, revealing tumor subtypes to be characterized by distinct mutation, methylation, and protein expression patterns. Additionally, previous genome-wide investigations have shown that aspirin or other non-steroidal anti-inflammatory drug use lowered CRC risk, particularly in the presence of 2 single-nucleotide polymorphisms (SNPs) on chromosome 12 and 15. Implementation of emerging screening strategies will require further determination of cost-effectiveness, as well as strong advocacy by public health departments to integrate new policies in communities at risk.

Hsu and colleagues[4] designed a model to determine CRC risk using common genetic susceptibility loci. In addition to sex, age, family history, and history of endoscopic examinations, the model took into consideration a genetic risk score (G-score) that was determined by 27 validated common CRC susceptibility loci identified from GWASs. The study demonstrated increased discriminatory accuracy from 0.51 to 0.59 ($P = .0028$) for men and 0.52 to 0.56 ($P = .14$) for women using their model compared with using family history alone, which reflects current CRC screening guidelines. Precision prevention aims to improve risk stratification by integrating genomic data to individually tailor starting age and interval for screening. Published in 2015, this study improved on similar risk-prediction models by increasing the number of CRC-associated common genetic variants for risk determination.

Determining Risk of Colorectal Cancer and Starting Age of Screening Based on Lifestyle, Environmental, and Genetic Factors

Current CRC guidelines are based on primarily based on age and family history. Additionally, there are a unique subset of patients that require specific screening, such as those with hereditary polyposis syndrome and inflammatory bowel disease. However, current CRC screening guidelines do not take into account the numerous known environmental risk factors or consider the growing body of CRC-associated genomic information. Jeon and colleagues[5] designed a model to determine CRC risk using 63 CRC-associated SNPs in addition to 19 lifestyle and environmental factors. Data were collected from 9748 CRC cases and 10,590 controls in the Genetics and Epidemiology of Colorectal Cancer Consortium and the Colorectal Transdisciplinary study, from 1992 through 2005. A total of 63 CRC-associated SNPs identified at 49 known CRC loci were previously identified by GWASs. A G-score was developed to account for the estimated strengths of CRC-association with each SNP. Similarly, a weighted environmental score was determined by 19 known environmental and lifestyle risk factors, including physical activity, alcohol consumption, and processed meat consumption. The study demonstrated increased discriminatory accuracy of 0.53 to 0.63 for men and 0.54 to 0.62 for women. Risk prediction models incorporating genetic and environmental risk factors provide an opportunity to improve risk stratification for screening recommendations compared with those relying on family history alone. A limitation of this study was that history of CRC endoscopic examination, which has a strong negative association with CRC risk, was not considered.

Personalized In Vitro and In Vivo Cancer Models to Guide Precision Medicine

To complement the genomic information and to provide therapeutic options for patients, Pauli and colleagues[6] integrated personalized patient-derived tumor organoids drug screens and patient-derived xenografts generation into their platform. A total of 145 specimens comprising 18 different tumor types derived from patients with metastatic solid tumors of epithelial and mesenchymal origin were collected. These included 10 tumors of the colon or rectum, among these tumors, 1 subject with stage IV colon cancer with mutations in KRAS and TP53, which was resistant to most agents, showed an exceptional response to the MEK inhibitor, trametinib, which was confirmed in organoid culture. A conditional screen with trametinib demonstrated the potential to combine this drug with several targeted agents. The combination screen for this subject showed that trametinib sensitized the KRAS mutant colon cancer cells to multiple FDA approved agents with little or no effect on their own (celecoxib, nilotinib, vorinostat, belinostat, and afatinib).

KRAS wild-type (WT) colorectal tumor cells from another subject with mutations in the APC gene, demonstrated sensitivity to epidermal growth factor receptor (EGFR) inhibitors, in particular afatinib. A sensitizing screen with the EGFR inhibitor afatinib, which was the highest scoring single agent, showed an enhanced response to histone deacetylase (HDAC) and Insulin-like Growth Factor-1 Receptor (IGF-1R) inhibitors.

They were thus able to identify unique combinations for individual subjects and showed that in vitro drug testing may identify effective therapeutic strategies and help guide the choice of appropriate clinical trials.

When personalized tumor cultures are not available to generate genomics to therapeutic responses, the alternate option can be to use data mining techniques with larger scale databases containing genomic data, functional drug profiles, clinical variables, and patient follow-up information.

PRECISION MEDICINE TRIALS FOR COLORECTAL CANCER

Most current precision medicine strategies for malignancies, including CRC, are based on DNA sequencing of archival or fresh tumor biopsies.

Tumor Characterization to Guide Experimental Targeted Therapy (TARGET) is a molecular profiling program with the primary aim to match patients with a broad range of advanced cancers to early-phase clinical trials based on analysis of both somatic mutations and copy number alterations across a 641 cancer-associated-gene panel in a single ctDNA assay.[7] In the first 100 TARGET subjects, ctDNA data showed good concordance with matched tumor. When a 2.5% variant allele frequency (VAF) threshold was used, actionable mutations were identified in 41 of 100 subjects, and 11 of these subjects received a matched therapy. Among other tumor types, this study looked at 23 CRCs, of which 74% were mutation positive, and average VAF in this group was 15.4% (range 3.4–65). The investigators concluded that the data support the application of ctDNA in early-phase trial settings.

Sicklick and colleagues[8] report on precision oncology trials based on molecular matching with predetermined monotherapies. Several of these trials have been hindered by very low matching rates (often 5%–10%) and low response rates. Low matching rates may be due to the use of limited gene panels, restrictive molecular matching algorithms, lack of drug availability, or the deterioration and death of end-stage patients before therapy can be implemented. A cross-institutional prospective study of Molecular Profile-Related Evidence to Determine Individualized Therapy for Advanced or Poor Prognosis Cancers (I-PREDICT, NCT02534675) was designed that used tumor DNA sequencing and timely therapeutic recommendations for individualized treatment with combination therapies. Targeting of a larger fraction of identified molecular alterations, yielding a higher matching score, correlated with significantly improved disease control rates and longer progression-free survival (PFS) and overall survival (OS) rates compared with patients in whom fewer somatic alterations were targeted. The most common primary tumor sites were gastrointestinal (eg, hepatopancreatobiliary) (42.2%). This high matching rate was based on several key factors: (1) molecular interrogation by Next-Generation Sequencing Testing (NGS) for a large panel of cancer-related genes, including assessment of tumor mutational burden, microsatellite instability (MSI) status, programmed death ligand 1 (PD-L1) immunohistochemistry, and ctDNA; (2) timely institutional molecular tumor board discussions, which occurred immediately on receipt of molecular results, including by ad hoc e-meetings, to inform treatment recommendations without delay; and (3) use of a medication acquisition specialist and clinical trials coordinator to ensure rapid access to drugs. Higher degrees of matching are associated with better outcomes than lower degrees of matching, and higher matching scores often require customized combinations, rather than single agents, as are often given in traditional precision oncology trials.

The investigators from the Worldwide Innovative Network (WIN) Association–WIN Consortium, conducted the WINTHER trial (NCT01856296) in which subjects were navigated to therapy based on fresh biopsy-derived DNA sequencing (arm A; 236 gene panel) or RNA expression (arm B; comparing tumor to normal).[9] Investigators from 5 countries in North America, Europe, and the Middle East were members of the clinical management committee. Of the 303 consented subjects, 107 subjects were evaluated for therapy (69 in arm A and 38 in arm B). An exploratory matching score (based on drugs administered) was assigned for all 107 evaluable subjects. They examined the use of tumor versus normal tissue as a comparator for transcriptomics. The level of basal gene expression was highly variable between individuals. Although the trial did not meet its primary endpoint for a PFS2 to PFS1 ratio of greater than 1.5, there were several novel paradigm shifts in the WINTHER trial that merit highlighting: (1) deployment of a transcriptomic arm (arm B) to navigate subjects with various solid tumors prospectively to a large panel of therapies, in addition to a genomic arm (arm A); (2) using a 236 NGS gene panel, rather than less comprehensive testing, for the genomic arm; (3) timely clinical management committee teleconference discussions that included investigators from centers in France, Spain, Israel, Canada, and the United States.

The WIN consortium trial used genomic or transcriptomic analysis to successfully match 35% of patients with refractory cancers from different countries despite varying drug and clinical trial resources. The WINTHER trial integrated a new generation of genomic and transcriptomic tools (a large panel NGS-based test and WINTHER RNA-based algorithms) in the decision-making process, but their interpretation by the physicians, cognizant of rapidly evolving knowledge, remained essential. The investigators concluded that genomic and transcriptomic profiling are both useful for improving therapy recommendations and patient outcome.

The National Cancer Institute's Molecular Analysis for Therapy Choice (NCI-MATCH) trial, the landmark precision medicine trial, released the results from several treatment arms, or substudies, of the trial. In May 2017, for the first time in history, the FDA approved an agent based purely on a mutation, without regard for tissue or site involved. The site-agnostic approval was granted to Merck's pembrolizumab (Keytruda) for adult and pediatric patients with unresectable or metastatic, microsatellite instability-high or mismatch repair-deficient solid tumors in the following scenarios: (1) progressed following prior treatment, (2) no satisfactory alternative treatment options, (3) Microsatellite instability – high (MSI-H) or mismatched repair-deficient (dMMR) CRC that had progressed following treatment with a fluoropyrimidine, oxaliplatin, and irinotecan.

Harris and colleagues[10] reported on the status of accrual from opening on August, 12, 2015, through July, 16, 2017, and expanded on future plans. The NCI-MATCH trial is the largest national study to date for patients with relapsed or refractory solid tumors, lymphomas, and myelomas, in which targeted therapy is based on individual tumor molecular alterations. The study noted that patients with dMMR may benefit from immune checkpoint inhibitor therapy secondary to increased mutational burden compared with mismatch repair (MMR)-proficient tumors.

Azad and colleagues[11] investigated whether nivolumab would be active in patients with noncolorectal dMMR cancers. The preliminary results of the first 35 enrolled (70% MLH1 (MutL homolog 1) loss, 30% MSH2 (MutS protein homolog 2) loss with minimum follow-up time of greater than 6 months was reported and the median prior therapies were 3. Common histologies included endometrioid endometrial (n = 10), prostate (n = 6), and breast (n = 3) cancer. Ten subjects remained on treatment, 7 stopped treatment due to adverse effects, 12 for disease progression. The overall response rate was 24% (8/33 subjects) with an additional 9 out of 33 (27%) subjects with stable disease. Three additional subjects had unconfirmed responses. Estimated 6-month PFS was 43% and median OS was not reached at this early time-point. Toxicity was predominantly low-grade. These results show that nivolumab has promising activity in mismatched repair-deficient non-CRCs.

PREDICTIVE BIOMARKERS AND THEIR USE IN COLORECTAL CANCER

Several key mutations are important in CRC initiation, progression, metastasis, and the response to some therapeutic agents. These mutations include APC (found in 80% of CRC tumors), TP53 (50%), KRAS (35%–45%), PIK3CA (20%–30%), and BRAF (10%), among others.[12] Each CRC has been shown to possess 2 to 6 driver mutations per tumor. To date, KRAS, NRAS, and BRAF mutations are used clinically because their presence predicts resistance to the anti-EGFR antibodies cetuximab and panitumumab.

Markowitz and Bertagnolli[13] reported on the molecular basis of individual susceptibility to CRC and to determine factors that initiate tumor development, progression, and responsiveness or resistance to antitumor agents. Loss of genomic stability can drive the development of CRC by facilitating the acquisition of multiple tumor-associated mutations. The most common type of genomic instability in CRC (80%–85% of sporadic CRCs) is chromosomal instability, an efficient mechanism for causing the physical loss of a WT copy of a tumor-suppressor gene, such as APC, P53, and SMAD family member 4 (SMAD4).

DNA mismatch-repair defects include germline defects such as hereditary non-polyposis colon cancer (HNPCC; primarily MLH1 and MSH2) that confer a 80% lifetime risk of CRC or germline inactivation of a base excision repair gene, mutY homologue (MUTYH, also called MYH). Patients with 2 inactive germline MYH alleles develop polyposis associated almost a 100% risk of CRC by 60 years of age. Mismatch-repair deficiency (MMR-d) cancers mainly arise in the proximal colon and involves inactivation of tumor-suppressor genes encoding TGF-BR2 (transforming growth factor b receptor type II) and BAX (BCL2-associated X protein). Aberrant MLH1 methylation and BRAF mutation are associated with the serrated-adenoma pathway.

Driver mutations impart a selective growth advantage to the cancer cell. Although this advantage is minor (0.4% increase) over many years this can result in a significant tumor size. The number of mutations is directly correlated with age with a 90-year-old patient having nearly twice the mutations compared to that in a 45-year-old patient.[14]

GWAS show varying types of genomic alterations including single-base substitutions, insertions, deletions, amplifications, homozygous deletions, and translocations. Driver mutations in CRC have about 3 to 6 mutations. In colon cancer, an average of 33 to 66 genes display subtle somatic mutations with about 95% being single-base substitutions.

Molecular profiling has become a pivotal component in guiding clinical decisions in metastatic colon cancer.[15] National Comprehensive Cancer Network (NCCN) guidelines recommend KRAS, NRAS, and BRAF mutation testing for all patients with metastatic CRC (mCRC). Patients with any known KRAS mutation (exon 2, 3, 4) or NRAS mutation (exon 2, 3, 4) should not be treated with either cetuximab or panitumumab. In patients with BRAF V600E mutation response to panitumumab or cetuximab is highly unlikely unless administered with a BRAF inhibitor. The testing can be performed on formalin-fixed paraffin-embedded tissue and either on primary CRCs or the metastasis.[16] All patients with KRAS, NRAS, or BRAF WT mCRC are candidates for treatment with anti-EGFR agents in combination FOLFOX or FOLFIRI as first line options. Regarding PIK3CA mutations, there are insufficient data to make any clear conclusion about their effect on response to anti-EGFR therapies. Activation of the PI3K signaling cascade can result in continued proliferative signaling independent of inhibition of EGFR. Continued efforts should be made to better understand the role of PIK3CA mutations in mCRC and its influence on treatment response.

With improved understanding of the role of biomarkers in treatment of CRC molecular profiling and treatment responses, there is higher likelihood of matching treatment options based on patient selection to improve outcomes.

CRC patients harboring wild-type KRAS are treated with anti-EGFR monoclonal antibodies such as cetuximab or panitumumab. Patient with poor response to this treatment likely have mutations in other genes like BRAF, PI3KCA, or PTEN in addition to KRAS. Lupini and colleagues[17] investigated a panel of 21 genes by parallel sequencing on the Ion Torrent Personal Genome Machine platform. They sequenced 65 CRCs (37 responsive and 28 resistant) that were treated with cetuximab or panitumumab. EGFR-pathway gene mutations (KRAS, NRAS, BRAF, PI3KCA) conferred resistance to therapy and were predictive of response (P = .001). Combined NRAS, BRAF and PIK3CA mutations were significantly associated with resistant phenotype (P = .045). Mutations in FBXW7 and SMAD4 were also present in cases that were nonresponsive to anti-EGFR moAb. Ability to predict treatment response increased with combining gene mutations with the exclusion of KRAS (P = .002) demonstrating the feasibility and benefit of multigene sequencing to assess response to therapy.

Although several resistance mechanisms have been identified, RAS mutational status is the only established predictive tumor biomarker for treatment of mCRC patients. RAS-activating mutations predict a lack treatment response, whereas low levels of primary resistance are observed in RAS WT patients (about 15%). However, even WT patients who initially respond to anti-EGFR therapy, eventually undergo tumor progression. Martins and colleagues[18] provided an overview on the mechanisms that contribute to resistance to EGFR-targeted therapy and highlight what is still missing in the understanding of these molecular mechanisms and approaches to overcome them.

The moAbs panitumumab and cetuximab target the EGFR and have proven value for the treatment of mCRC. EGFR-mediated signaling involves 2 main intracellular cascades: KRAS activates BRAF, which in turn triggers the mitogen-activated protein kinases. On the other hand, membrane localization of the lipid kinase PIK3CA counteracts PTEN and promotes AKT1 phosphorylation, thereby activating a parallel intracellular mechanism. Constitutive activation of KRAS bypasses the corresponding signaling cascade; therefore, patients with KRAS-mutated mCRC are clinically resistant to therapy with panitumumab or cetuximab. Sartore-Bianchi and colleagues[19] hypothesized that mutations activating PIK3CA could also influence responsiveness to EGFR-targeted moAbs through a similar mechanism. They performed mutational analysis of PIK3CA and KRAS, and evaluation of the PTEN protein status, in 110 subjects with mCRC treated with anti-EGFR moAbs. They observed 15 (13.6%) PIK3CA and 32 (29.0%) KRAS mutations. PIK3CA mutations were significantly associated with clinical resistance to panitumumab or cetuximab; none of the mutated subjects achieved objective response (P = .038). When only KRAS WT tumors were analyzed, the statistical correlation was even stronger (P = .016). Subjects with PIK3CA mutations displayed inferior PFS (P = .035). This study showed that PIK3CA mutations can independently influence therapeutic response to panitumumab or cetuximab in mCRC. When the molecular status of the PIK3CA-PTEN and KRAS pathways are concomitantly determined, up to 70% of mCRC subjects who are unlikely to respond to EGFR moAbs could be identified.

The Evaluation of Genomic Applications in Practice and Prevention Working Group (EWG)[20] revealed a high level of evidence to recommend clinical use of KRAS mutation analysis to predict benefit from treatment with cetuximab or panitumumab in patients with mCRC. Insufficient evidence was found to recommend testing for mutations in

NRAS or PIK3CA, or loss of expression of PTEN or AKT proteins. There was insufficient evidence to recommend BRAF V600E mutation testing.

Mutation testing for KRAS exon 2 is used for patient selection in WT mCRC tumors for treatment with cetuximab and panitumumab. Therkildsen and colleagues[21] reviewed the impact of alterations in KRAS (outside of exon 2), NRAS, BRAF, PIK3CA, and PTEN on the clinical benefit derived from anti-EGFR treatment. A meta-analysis of 22 studies including 2395 subjects showed that mutations in KRAS exons 3 and 4, BRAF, PIK3CA, and nonfunctional PTEN significantly predicted poor objective response rates and thereby resistance to anti-EGFR therapies.. Mutations in KRAS exons 3 and 4 were associated with shorter progression free survival (hazard ratio [HR] 2.19), similar results were noted in mutations in NRAS (HR 1.85), BRAF (HR 2.52), PIK3CA (HR 1.43), and alterations in PTEN (HR 2.09). They suggested analysis of biomarkers beyond KRAS exon 2 for prediction of clinical benefit from anti-EGFR antibodies in mCRC.

The RAS-MAPK and PI3K signaling pathways are important in tumorigenesis. The BRAF, KRAS, and PI3KCA genes code 3 partners of this network and are activated by mutations in CRC. Barault and colleagues[22] evaluated the prognosis of subjects with activated-network colonic adenocarcinomas in a population-based study. Colonic adenocarcinomas were evaluated for BRAF, KRAS, and PI3KCA gene mutations. After adjusting for age and microsatellite instability, network activation by mutation of at least one of these genes was significantly associated with female gender (P = .02) and proximal tumor location (P< .001). Lower 3-year survival was noted with network activation by mutation of at least 1 gene that persisted on multivariate analysis after adjusting for sex, age, tumor location, stage, and micro satellite instability (HR 1.48, 95% CI 1.07–2.04). The clinical and therapeutic value of evaluating mutations within the signaling network was emphasized by this study.

De Roock and colleagues[23] analyzed 1022 tumor DNA samples (73 from fresh-frozen and 949 from formalin-fixed, paraffin-embedded tissue) from subjects treated with cetuximab between 2001 and 2008 that were gathered from 11 centers in 7 European countries. A total of 773 primary tumor samples had sufficient quality DNA and were included in mutation frequency analyses; mass spectrometry genotyping of tumor samples for KRAS, BRAF, NRAS, and PIK3CA was done centrally. Objective response, PFS, and OS in molecularly defined subgroups of the 649 chemotherapy-refractory subjects treated with cetuximab plus chemotherapy were studied. Of these, 40.0% of the tumors harbored a KRAS mutation, 14.5% had a PIK3CA mutation (of which most, 68.5%, were located in exon 9 and 20.4% in exon 20), 4.7% harbored a BRAF mutation, and 2.6% had an NRAS mutation. KRAS mutants did not derive benefit compared with WTs, with a response rate of 6.7% versus 35.8% (OR 0.13, 95% CI 0.07–0.22, P<.0001), a median PFS of 12 weeks versus 24 weeks (HR 1.98, 95% CI 1.66–2.36, P<.0001), and a median OS of 32 weeks versus 50 weeks (HR 1.75, 95% CI 1.47–2.09, P<.0001). In KRAS WTs, carriers of BRAF and NRAS mutations had a significantly lower response rate than did BRAF and NRAS WTs, with a response rate of 8.3 versus 38.0%, respectively (OR 0.15, 95% CI 0.02–0.51, P = .0012). Higher response rates of 38.1% were noted in NRAS WTs versus 7.7% in carriers of NRAS mutations (OR 0.14, 95% CI 0.007–0.70, P = .013). PIK3CA exon 9 mutations had no effect, whereas exon 20 mutations were associated with a worse outcome compared with WTs, with a 0% response rate and lower median PFS and OS. Multivariate analysis and conditional inference trees confirmed that, if KRAS is not mutated, assessing BRAF, NRAS, and PIK3CA exon 20 mutations (in that order) gives additional information about outcome. BRAF, NRAS, and PIK3CA exon 20 mutations were significantly associated with a low response rate. Objective response rates could be improved by additional genotyping of BRAF, NRAS, and PIK3CA exon 20 mutations in a KRAS WT population.

ONCOGENIC MUTATIONS AS PREDICTIVE FACTORS IN COLORECTAL CANCER

The Epidermal Growth Factor Receptor (EGFR), is an important therapeutic target in mCRC.[24] An activation of several pathways downstream of EGFR, including the RAS-MAPK and PI3K-AKT pathways, and also the PLC, STAT, and SRC-FAK pathways, have been shown to be a key event in tumor proliferation, angiogenesis, and cell survival. The anti-EGFR moAbs cetuximab and panitumumab have been demonstrated to be valuable therapeutic options for mCRC. However, their efficacy remains modest with reported objective response rates between 8% to 23%. Lièvre and colleagues[24] reviewed mechanisms of resistance to anti-EGFR antibodies used by tumors. In a study of mCRC subjects, the investigators showed a relationship between the presence of tumor KRAS mutations and lack of response to cetuximab.

Oncogenic activation of intracellular signaling pathways downstream of EGFR has a major role in colorectal carcinogenesis but has also been reported to be an important mechanism of resistance to anti-EGFR antibodies.[24] 40% of activating mutations inCRCs are KRAS mutations and are a major predictive marker of resistance to anti-EGFR antibodies. BRAF or PIK3CA mutations, or loss of PTEN expression might be predictive of anti-EGFR moAbs response but require further studies before being incorporated in clinical practice. Understanding these markers of resistance to anti-EGFR therapy will allow development of new therapies that can target escape mechanisms used by tumors to circumvent a pathway that has been pharmacologically blocked by anti-EGFR.

The BRAF inhibitors (vemurafenib and dabrafenib) and MEK inhibitor (trametinib) were approved for patients with melanoma bearing BRAF pV600E mutation, and anti-EGFR moAbs (cetuximab and panitumumab) for CRC without RAS mutations. EGFR tyrosine kinase inhibitors (gefitinib and erlotinib) targeting certain EGFR mutations for non-small cell lung cancers (NSCLCs) and ALK tyrosine kinase inhibitor (crizotinib) for NSCLC carrying the ALK gene translocations.[25] Molecular testing of targeted mutations has become essential to select patients for these therapies. Numerous potential biomarkers are being investigated to explore meaningful targets for clinical management of cancers. However, so far, only a limited number have been proven to be clinically meaningful and, subsequently, become or potentially become part of standard patient care.

Guidelines for Biomarker Testing

Universal or reflex testing, has been recommended for CRC and this has been endorsed by the EWG at the Centers for Disease Control and Prevention, the American Society for Clinical Pathology, College of American Pathologists, Association for Molecular Pathology, and American Society of Clinical Oncology. The US Multi-Society Task Force on Colorectal Cancer and American Gastroenterological Association also recommends universal genetic testing of tumors of all newly diagnosed CRC patients. The NCCN Colon and Rectal Cancer Panel endorses universal MMR or MSI testing of all patients with a personal history of colon or rectal cancer to identify individuals with Lynch syndrome,[16] which is relevant for treatment selection in stage IV disease.

Secondary Prevention Studies in Colorectal Cancer

Use of aspirin after diagnosis of CRC is associated with improved survival. In the Eindhoven Cancer Registry, 599 patients with CRC were analyzed for BRAF and KRAS mutation status and compared to data on aspirin use (80 mg) taken from the PHARMO Database Network. Improved OS was noted in BRAF WT tumors (RR of 0.60, 95% CI.24 0.44–0.83)[26] but not in patients with BRAF-mutated tumors. The effect of aspirin on survival was not influenced by KRAS mutational status. Low-dose aspirin use after CRC diagnosis was associated with improved survival in BRAF WT tumors only. Understanding the CRC subtypes responding to aspirin treatment might help in the development of personalized treatment regimens.

SUMMARY

There have been significant advances in the development of precision medicine for colorectal carcinoma influencing areas of screening, treatment, and potentially prevention. Advances in molecular techniques have made it possible for better patient selection for therapies and it is important that mutational analysis be performed at the time of diagnosis to guide treatment. Future efforts should focus on validating these treatments in specific subgroups of colorectal tumors and gaining deeper understanding of the mechanisms of resistance to therapies. This will subsequently enable treatment optimization, promote efficacy, and reduce treatment costs and toxicities.

REFERENCES

1. American Cancer Society. Cancer facts & figures 2019. Atlanta (GA): American Cancer Society; 2019. Available at: https://www.cancer.org/content/dam/cancer-org/research/cancer-facts-and-statistics/annual-cancer-facts-and-figures/2019/cancer-facts-and-figures-2019.pdfLast. Accessed August 29, 2019.
2. Loomans-Kropp HA, Umar A. Cancer prevention and screening: the next step in the era of precision medicine. NPJ Precis Oncol 2019;3:3.
3. Stewart BW, Bray F, Forman D, et al. Cancer prevention as part of precision medicine: 'plenty to be done. Carcinogenesis 2016;37(1):2–9.
4. Hsu L, Jeon J, Brenner H, et al. A model to determine colorectal cancer risk using common genetic susceptibility loci. Gastroenterology 2015;148(7):1330–9.e14.
5. Jeon J, Du M, Schoen RE, et al. Determining risk of colorectal cancer and starting age of screening based on lifestyle, environmental, and genetic factors. Gastroenterology 2018;154(8):2152–64.e19.
6. Pauli C, Hopkins BD, Prandi D, et al. Personalized in vitro and in vivo cancer models to guide precision medicine. Cancer Discov 2017;7(5):462–77.
7. Rothwell DG, Ayub M, Cook N, et al. Utility of ctDNA to support patient selection for early phase clinical trials: the TARGET study. Nat Med 2019;25(5):738–43.
8. Sicklick JK, Kato S, Okamura R, et al. Molecular profiling of cancer patients enables personalized combination therapy: the I-PREDICT study. Nat Med 2019;25(5):744–50.
9. Rodon J, Soria J-C, Berger R, et al. Genomic and transcriptomic profiling expands precision cancer medicine: the WINTHER trial. Nat Med 2019;25(5):751–8.

10. Harris L, Chen A, O'Dwyer P, et al: Update on the NCI-molecular analysis for therapy choice (NCI-MATCH/EAY131) precision medicine trial. 2017 AACR-NCI-EORTC International Conference on Molecular Targets and Cancer Therapeutics. Abstract B080. Philadelphia. Presented October 29, 2017.

11. Azad N, Overman M, Gray R, et al. Nivolumab in mismatch-repair deficient (MMR-d) cancers: NCI-MATCH Trial (Molecular Analysis for Therapy Choice) arm Z1D preliminary results. J Immunother Cancer 2017;5(Suppl 3): O37. Presented at the 32nd Annual Meeting and Pre-Conference Programs of the Society for Immunotherapy of Cancer (SITC 2017): Late-Breaking Abstracts.

12. Mohapatra SS, Batra SK, Bharadwaj S, et al. Precision medicine for CRC patients in the veteran population: state-of-the-art, challenges and research directions. Dig Dis Sci 2018;63(5):1123–38.

13. Markowitz SD, Bertagnolli MM. Molecular origins of cancer: molecular basis of colorectal cancer. N Engl J Med 2009;361(25):2449–60.

14. Vogelstein B, Papadopoulos N, Velculescu VE, et al. Cancer genome landscapes. Science 2013;339(6127):1546–58.

15. Tran NH, Cavalcante LL, Lubner SJ, et al. Precision medicine in colorectal cancer: the molecular profile alters treatment strategies. Ther Adv Med Oncol 2015;7(5):252–62.

16. NCCN Clinical Practice Guidelines in Oncology (NCCN Guidelines) Colon Cancer Version 3.2019. https://www.nccn.org/professionals/physician_gls/pdf/colon_blocks.pdf. Accessed October 14, 2019.

17. Lupini L, Bassi C, Mlcochova J, et al. Prediction of response to anti-EGFR antibody-based therapies by multigene sequencing in colorectal cancer patients. BMC Cancer 2015;15:808.

18. Martins M, Mansinho A, Cruz-Duarte R, et al. Anti-EGFR therapy to treat metastatic colorectal cancer: not for all. Adv Exp Med Biol 2018;1110:113–31.

19. Sartore-Bianchi A, Martini M, Molinari F, et al. PIK3CA mutations in colorectal cancer are associated with clinical resistance to EGFR-targeted monoclonal antibodies. Cancer Res 2009;69(5):1851–7.

20. Calonge N, Fisher NL, Berg AO, et al. Evaluation of Genomic Applications in Practice and Prevention (EGAPP) Working Group. Recommendations from the EGAPP Working Group: can testing of tumor tissue for mutations in EGFR pathway downstream effector genes in patients with metastatic colorectal cancer improve health outcomes by guiding decisions regarding anti-EGFR therapy? Genet Med 2013;15(7):517–27.

21. Therkildsen C, Bergmann TK, Henrichsen-Schnack T, et al. The predictive value of KRAS, NRAS, BRAF, PIK3CA and PTEN for anti-EGFR treatment in metastatic colorectal cancer: a systematic review and meta-analysis. Acta Oncol 2014; 53(7):852–64.

22. Barault L, Veyrie N, Jooste V, et al. Mutations in the RAS-MAPK, PI(3)K (phosphatidylinositol-3-OH kinase) signaling network correlate with poor survival in a population-based series of colon cancers. Int J Cancer 2008; 122(10):2255–9.

23. De Roock W, Claes B, Bernasconi D, et al. Effects of KRAS, BRAF, NRAS, and PIK3CA mutations on the efficacy of cetuximab plus chemotherapy in chemotherapy-refractory metastatic colorectal cancer: a retrospective consortium analysis. Lancet Oncol 2010;11(8):753–62.

24. Lièvre A, Blons H, Laurent-Puig P. Oncogenic mutations as predictive factors in colorectal cancer. Oncogene 2010;29(21):3033–43.

25. Sandhu J, Lavingia V, Fakih M. Systemic treatment for metastatic colorectal cancer in the era of precision medicine. J Surg Oncol 2019; 119(5):564–82.
26. Frouws MA, Reimers MS, Swets M, et al. The influence of BRAF and KRAS mutation status on the association between aspirin use and survival after colon cancer diagnosis. PLoS One 2017;12(1):e0170775.

Genomics and the History of Precision Oncology

Deborah B. Doroshow, MD, PhD[a], James H. Doroshow, MD[b],*

KEYWORDS

- Basket trial • Bucket trial • Master protocol • Cancer drug development
- Precision oncology

KEY POINTS

- The use of molecular tumor characteristics to select systemic therapy for individual patients has grown dramatically over the past 20 years.
- The identification of tumoral DNA abnormalities using rapid gene sequencing techniques has underpinned the discovery of treatments for certain patients independent of disease histology.
- Clinical trial designs using the master protocol concept have facilitated the simultaneous evaluation of multiple new therapies based on matching drugs to specific genomic abnormalities.

INTRODUCTION

The use of molecular characterization of an individual patient's tumor in routine oncologic practice began only 20 years ago. In that short time, it has enhanced the specificity and efficacy of cancer therapy.[1] Molecular selection criteria, both genomic and protein based, have now been used to support the first histology-independent US Food and Drug Administration (FDA) approvals of anticancer agents.[2–7] This paradigmatic shift in oncologic practice has been accompanied by discontinuation of nonspecific cytotoxic anticancer agent development.[8]

The use of precision medicine principles in cancer therapy[9] depends on measurement of biologic characteristics in a tumor that suggest the potential value of a specific molecularly targeted treatment. This shift away from nonspecific mechanisms of tumor cell killing has occurred because of improvements in biomarker discovery

Disclosure Statement: D.B. Doroshow does consulting for Boehringer Ingelheim, Ipsen. J.H. Doroshow has nothing to disclose. The article is supported by ZIA BC 011078; Phase 0/1 Clinical Trials from the National Cancer Institute (JHD); ASCO Young Investigator Award (DBD).
[a] Department of Medicine and Cancer Center, Icahn School of Medicine at Mount Sinai, 1 Gustave Levy Place, New York, NY 10029, USA; [b] Division of Cancer Treatment and Diagnosis, National Cancer Institute, NIH, Suite 3A44, Building 31, 31 Center Drive, Bethesda, MD 20892, USA
* Corresponding author.
E-mail address: doroshoj@mail.nih.gov

and validation, and the availability of instrumentation capable of previously inconceivable levels of diagnostic throughput. Precision oncology has also advanced because of innovations in clinical trial design.[10–12]

Although precision oncology has changed both the landscape of treatment options for patients with cancer and the fabric of clinical and translational research, cytotoxic agents remain the backbone of therapy for the majority of cancers, and targeted agents rarely provide durable responses. Moreover, innovative clinical trial designs to evaluate novel targets remain in the early stages of development, engendering numerous operational challenges[11] and modest clinical benefit to date.[12,13] This article examines the history of precision oncology, including milestone developments in therapeutics, translational science, and clinical trial design over the last 20 years.

Several case studies illustrate the benefits and limitations of the so-called one gene, one drug, one disease paradigm. Although clinical responses may be common and dramatic, they are rarely lasting. Moreover, this model does not apply to the majority of neoplastic diseases. These case studies also illustrate the ways in which targeted therapies have unexpected effects and frequently transform the natural history of disease. The identification and targeting of molecular aberrations requires sufficiently efficient and accurate technologies, many of which have become more sensitive and comprehensive over the last 10 years. Finally, master protocols have been developed to provide a coordinated framework for evaluation of multiple therapeutic approaches in 1 or more molecularly defined tumor types, with the goal of improving the efficiency of the cancer clinical trials process. Such studies can be designed to provide sufficient information to support an application for new drug approval by the FDA, or, more frequently, to identify biomarker-selected drugs that can be more effectively predicted to be successful in the setting of a subsequent, definitive randomized study.

THE MAGIC BULLET PARADIGM IN PRECISION ONCOLOGY, 2000 TO 2010

Most retellings of the beginnings of precision oncology focus on the development of a series of drugs, each of which was intended to treat a single tumor type with a single molecular aberration. Each were heralded by physicians and by the lay public as near miracles of science. Although these developments were critical to the development of precision oncology, they were often unpredictable and uniformly never sudden. We discuss them here not as a means of uncritically listing a series of successes, but as a window into the promises and limitations of precision oncology more broadly.

In the late 1980s, Dennis Slamon and his colleagues at the University of California, Los Angeles demonstrated that one-quarter of breast cancers could be characterized by amplification or overexpression of human epidermal growth factor-2 (HER2), a tyrosine kinase receptor, which activates multiple signal transduction pathways to regulate cell growth.[14,15] Moreover, patients harboring such tumors had a poorer prognosis than those who did not.[14,15] Simultaneously, multiple investigators determined that HER2 overexpression induced tumorigenesis, making the protein a desirable therapeutic target.[16–18] A humanized HER2 antibody, engineered at Genentech (South San Francisco, CA) in 1992,[19] was quickly introduced into multiple phase I and phase II clinical trials, the latter of which focused on enrolling only patients with increased HER2 expression by immunohistochemistry.[20] However, the definition of increased HER2 expression was inconsistent; 1 trial enrolled patients with 25% or greater membrane staining, a second enrolled those whose tumors had "light to strong" immunohistochemical staining, and a third used the now-standard 2+/3+ nomenclature to refer to weak or complete tumor cell membrane staining in more than 10% of cells.[20]

Despite modest activity in a placebo-controlled phase III study (using the latter definition of HER2 positivity) trastuzumab (Herceptin) was approved by the FDA in 1998.[21] Trastuzumab was hailed by the popular press as "ushering in a new era of cancer treatment that attempts to target the very flawed genetic mechanisms that cause the disease."[22] The *Washington Post* described how 1 patient's impending death was dramatically reversed by trastuzumab, which shrunk her liver metastases "to mere dots" and showed "how 20 years of basic cancer research are beginning to pay off for patients."[23] Yet the popular press also reminded readers that although trastuzumab seems to be a wonder drug, it was not a cure.[22]

Although trastuzumab did not dramatically improve outcomes as a single agent, it has become a critical, life-prolonging adjunct to chemotherapy in the metastatic,[24] neoadjuvant,[25] and adjuvant[26] settings. The identification of HER2 as a valuable therapeutic target spurred additional work resulting in the development of trastuzumab emtansine, a novel antibody–drug conjugate targeting HER2,[27] and pertuzumab, a monoclonal antibody binding a different epitope of HER2.[28] Perhaps most intriguingly, trastuzumab has changed the natural history of HER2-positive breast cancer. Whereas Slamon and colleagues initially identified HER2 overexpression as a poor prognostic marker, patients who are treated with HER2-directed therapies may no longer be at a survival disadvantage. Now, HER2 overexpression has become a predictive biomarker, indicative of a subset of patients likely to respond to HER2-directed therapy.

Three years after trastuzumab was approved by the FDA, another landmark drug was introduced: imatinib for the treatment of chronic myeloid leukemia (CML). The press similarly described the drug as a magic bullet, proclaiming that "the dream of a pill that can treat cancer with almost no side effects became a reality" and referring to targeted drugs as "smart bombs" that did not induce the collateral damage seen with cytotoxic chemotherapy.[29] Patients who had participated in clinical trials spread the news in online chat rooms before trial results had even been published.[30] This enthusiasm was understandable. The phase I study of imatinib, a small molecule inhibitor of the BCR-ABL tyrosine kinase, had identified no maximally tolerated dose, and 53 of 54 patients achieved a complete hematologic response[31]; based on these results as well as those of 3 phase II studies, imatinib was granted accelerated approval by the FDA in 2001. The 72 days required for FDA review was the fastest agency approval in the history of anticancer agent development.[32]

Despite the perception of a sudden breakthrough, the story of imatinib illustrates the lengthy research timeframe involved in identifying a molecular target and crafting a drug to engage it. Although CML had been described as a disease entity in Germany and Scotland in 1845,[33] the majority of work done to identify the *BCR-ABL* fusion as the causative aberration in CML was performed between 1960 and 1990.[34] In 1960, Peter Nowell and David Hungerford described a "minute chromosome" present in the peripheral blood of 7 patients with what was then known as chronic granulocytic leukemia.[35] In the early 1970s, Caspersson and colleagues[36] and O'Riordan and colleagues[37] identified the abnormally small chromosome as number 22 using novel quinacrine mustard fluorescence techniques, and Janet Rowley[38] described its balanced translocation with the long arm of chromosome 9. In the 1970s and 1980s, work with retroviruses was critical to the identification of multiple putative oncogenes; one of these was c-abl, the human cellular homologue of the Abelson murine leukemia virus, which was translocated from 9q to the breakpoint cluster region (BCR) of 22q-in patients with CML.[34] In the mid-1980s, Davis and colleagues[39] and Ben-Neriah and colleagues[40] discovered that the resulting chimeric messenger RNA transcript was itself a tyrosine kinase, and murine work published by Daley and colleagues[41] and Heisterkamp and colleagues[42] in 1990 identified the *BCR-ABL* translocation as necessary and sufficient to induce CML.

Thus, by 1990, the *BCR-ABL* oncogene had been established as universally causative in CML; hence, the resulting tyrosine kinase was an attractive therapeutic target. Yet, general skepticism remained regarding the feasibility of inhibiting tyrosine kinases, with regard to the specificity, toxicity, and efficacy of doing so in heterogeneous cancers.[34] High-throughput screens of chemical libraries identified the 2-phenylaminopyrimidines as promising inhibitors of BCR-ABL in the early 1990s, and by 1996 Brian Druker and colleagues had published in vitro and in vivo data demonstrating that one such agent—STI571, or imatinib—potently inhibited the BCR-ABL kinase and killed CML cells.[34] Five years later, STI571 had been approved by the FDA. Although the development of imatinib had itself been brisk, the identification of BCR-ABL as a therapeutic target was an effort spanning more than 3 decades, an element of the imatinib story that is easy to overlook.[34]

The history of imatinib has been unusual in other ways, one of which is the durability of the responses produced by the drug. Resistance to therapy does develop and has spurred the introduction of second- and third-line agents. Still, patients with CML who are treated with BCR-ABL tyrosine kinase inhibitors can expect to live near-normal lifespans.[43] The introduction of these drugs, 5 of which are now FDA approved, has altered the natural history of CML to the extent that the field is now exploring the potential of therapy discontinuation.[44]

Although the importance of identifying a molecular target before developing a relevant therapy may seems to be obvious, in many prominent cases a target has been identified and refined during the course of drug development. For the epidermal growth factor receptor (EGFR), similar developments occurred in the development of EGFR-targeted agents in both lung and colorectal cancers. Initial work on EGFR, which was known to play an important role in modulating proliferative cell signaling, was based on its overexpression in multiple tumor types, including non-small cell lung cancer (NSCLC).[45] However, phase I trials of the EGFR tyrosine kinase inhibitor gefitinib produced few clinical responses.[46–48] Two phase II studies of gefitinib in NSCLC were slightly more promising, with response rates of 9% to 19%.[49,50] However, a retrospective analysis of tumor specimens from these 2 trials found no relationship between EGFR expression (as determined by immunohistochemistry) and clinical response.[51] Based on the results of these trials, gefitinib was granted accelerated approval by the FDA in 2003.[52] However, review by the FDA also noted the negative, unpublished results of 2 phase III studies that failed to show clinical benefit of gefitinib in combination with chemotherapy in patients with advanced NSCLC.[52–54]

Several groups of investigators sought to characterize responders further by analyzing tumor specimens from patients entered in phase II studies as well as those treated during expanded access programs. They identified several subgroups of patients with higher response rates: Japanese patients (compared with non-Japanese patients),[50] women,[49,55] never smokers,[56,57] and patients with adenocarcinoma histologies.[55–57] Simultaneously, several groups of investigators sequenced the *EGFR* gene in lung cancer specimens from patients who had been treated with gefitinib on clinical trials. They identified mutations in the *EGFR* tyrosine kinase domain in almost all tumors from patients who had responded, which were not present in nonresponders, establishing mutated *EGFR*—not overexpressed EGFR—as the molecular target for gefitinib.[57–59]

Although EGFR-targeted therapies have become a success story in lung cancer, their evolving history is more representative of targeted therapies than that of imatinib, in that resistance to treatment is inevitable. Over the last 10 years, studies have focused on the development of second- and third-generation EGFR inhibitors that specifically target mechanisms of resistance to first generation inhibitors such as the T790M mutation in exon 21 of *EGFR*.[60–64] Currently, the effort to characterize mechanisms of resistance to third generation inhibitors is ongoing with the aim of developing therapies that target these alterations or prevent their emergence.[65] Patients starting first-line osimertinib, a third-generation EGFR tyrosine kinase inhibitor, may respond for up to 22 months.[66] However, upon progression they are faced with the options of cytotoxic chemotherapy and immune checkpoint inhibitors, the latter of which have decreased efficacy in *EGFR* mutant NSCLC.[67–69]

Although resistance to targeted therapies may be due to so-called on-target molecular alterations, such as additional EGFR mutations, it often results from compensatory mechanisms, especially when a target is one member of a signaling pathway. This type of resistance proved an early stumbling block in the development of cetuximab, a competitive inhibitor of the extracellular domain of EGFR. Similar to gefitinib, cetuximab was studied in colon cancer based on the premise that EGFR was overexpressed in the majority of colorectal cancers, as well as promising preclinical data in colorectal cancer models.[70] The first phase III study of cetuximab, which studied it alone and in combination with irinotecan, used this rationale and required evidence of immunohistochemical expression of EGFR to enroll.[71] Seeking to better characterize cetuximab responders and nonresponders only a few years later, 2 French groups screened the tumors of clinical trial participants for mutations in *KRAS*, which was involved in EGFR downstream signaling. Not only did mutated *KRAS* predict for resistance to cetuximab, zero patients who responded to cetuximab had tumors with a *KRAS* mutation,[72–74] a finding confirmed in a larger retrospective study performed by a group from Australia and Canada.[4] Extended RAS testing is now recommended to demonstrate that a tumor is truly wild type before treating a patient with cetuximab to predict primary resistance.[75]

It is now clear that downstream resistance accounts for a substantial proportion of acquired resistance to targeted therapies, a lesson learned in the development of BRAF inhibitors for patients with metastatic melanoma. Although the BRAF inhibitors vemurafenib and dabrafenib both improved progression-free survival (PFS) in patients with untreated *BRAF*[V600E] mutated advanced melanoma compared with chemotherapy in 2 phase III studies, responses were short lived, with a median PFS of just over 5 months for both drugs.[76,77] Additional pharmacodynamic studies performed on patient tumor specimens from these and other trials found that acquired resistance to BRAF inhibitors was frequently associated with upregulation of signaling in the downstream MAPK pathway.[78–80] As a result, combinations of BRAF and MEK inhibitors were studied in multiple large phase III trials and were found to improve both PFS and overall survival compared with the use of BRAF inhibitors alone[81–84]; these combinations now comprise the standard of care therapy for patients with *BRAF*-mutated melanoma. These cases clearly demonstrate both the promise and the limitations of the magic bullet model of precision oncology, and have more recently led to efforts to identify promising combinations of targeted therapies.[85]

THE PROMISE AND LIMITATIONS OF TUMOR PROFILING

To detect molecular alterations that can be targeted, reliable and efficient technology is required. The early work on trastuzumab was limited to immunohistochemical staining, whereas fluorescent in situ hybridization is now a routine component of HER2 testing for tumor samples that demonstrate equivocal (2+) immunohistochemical staining; this combined approach has changed the definition of HER2-positive tumors.[86] In the 2000s and early 2010s, molecular alterations could be detected using either immunohistochemical evaluations of protein expression or PCR-based evaluations of mutational hotspots, which could miss uncommon alterations. In 2019, a patient's tumor may undergo high throughput massively parallel DNA and RNA sequencing (often referred to as next-generation sequencing) over a matter of 2 or 3 weeks to identify potential therapeutic targets.[87,88] These analyses, which may examine several hundred genes or even comprise whole exome or whole genome sequencing, are regularly performed on the tumors of patients treated at tertiary cancer centers and in the community. The latter was made more accessible owing to the recent announcement from the Centers for Medicare and Medicaid Services that Medicare will cover next-generation tumor profiling for patients with advanced cancer.[89]

Genomic and proteomic analyses now have the capacity to detect a variety of aberrations beyond point mutations, including insertion and deletion mutations, copy number alterations, chromosomal rearrangements, gene fusions, DNA methylation patterns, transcript levels, and levels of protein expression.[88] Analysis of a patient's tumor is often paired with an evaluation of matched normal cells, most often from a buccal swab or peripheral blood, to distinguish somatic aberrations found only in a tumor from germline abnormalities.[90] More recently, examinations of circulating tumor cells and circulating tumor DNA have been investigated as a means of dynamically and noninvasively assessing tumor burden as well as evaluating the changing genomic landscape of a tumor throughout a patient's treatment, with an eye to better understanding the mechanisms of drug resistance.[91–93]

These advances have enabled the detection of low frequency alterations and have fostered the development of many new targeted therapies. However, complex challenges remain. Tumor profiling reports may list the molecular aberrations identified in a patient's tumor, but only a minority at best may be targetable with approved or experimental agents. Such reports may neglect to describe the allelic frequency of such aberrations or distinguish between driver mutations—those which induce tumorigenesis—and passenger mutations, which are not themselves pathogenic.[88,94,95] Moreover, tumor heterogeneity may limit the applicability of these findings.[96,97] As in the case of BRAF inhibition in metastatic melanoma, efforts to target tumor molecular aberrations have been hampered by the almost universal development of on- or off-target resistance.[94] This has led to a recent focus on evaluating combinations of agents to delay the emergence of such resistance, for example, by inhibiting a signaling pathway at more than 1 level.[81]

NOVEL METHODS FOR EVALUATING TARGETED THERAPIES USING MASTER PROTOCOLS

Although technologies like next-generation sequencing have facilitated the detection of targetable molecular alterations, novel clinical trial designs—many of which are still in the early phases of development—have become critical to testing targeted agents. In the early 2010s, investigations of exceptional responders to targeted therapies were common.[98] In other instances, a patient's response to a therapy that had been matched to a specific tumor alteration was compared with that patient's response to a previous standard of care agent.[99] Many academic cancer centers developed molecular tumor boards in which a group of experts reviewed the molecular alterations in a patient's tumor and recommended a matched FDA-approved therapy, an off-label standard therapy, or a clinical trial.[6,87] Such tumor boards are increasingly common in both the academic and community settings.

In efforts to evaluate the concept of precision oncology more broadly, several studies have attempted to assess whether matched therapy provides greater clinical benefit than standard-of-care therapy. Multiple single-institution, observational studies have shown that it is feasible to match patients to both standard and investigational therapies, and that doing so may improve clinical outcomes. However, only a minority of patients could be assigned a matched therapy, and none of the trials were randomized.[100–104] SHIVA, the first randomized trial of precision oncology as an approach, randomized patients with multiple tumor histologies to receive either 1 of 11 molecularly targeted agents based on the presence or absence of aberrations in the hormone receptor, phosphoinositide 3-kinase/AKT/mammalian target of rapamycin, and RAF/MEK pathways or physician's choice of standard therapy.[105] Although no difference in PFS was observed, the study used only a limited range of targeted therapies and did not account for differing levels of evidence regarding the relevance of each patient's pathway aberration.

Master protocols, which permit the testing of patients with multiple tumor histologies and/or tumor molecular aberrations, are both powerful and complex frameworks used to test a variety of hypotheses simultaneously. By grouping tumors by molecular alteration, they move oncology toward a less histology based and more molecularly based diagnostic and clinical framework.[13] Classically, master protocols have been described as falling into 1 of 2 categories: basket studies, which seek to treat patients across multiple histologies whose tumors share the same alteration, and umbrella studies, which assign patients with 1 tumor type to one of several therapies based on tumor profiling data.[13] Although such studies may be used for FDA registration of a new agent, they are more often signal-finding trials intended to identify potentially interesting therapies worthy of further study in certain patient populations.

Basket studies play a critical role in promoting a histology-agnostic approach to treating cancer. Two phase II studies of pembrolizumab, an anti-programmed death 1 antibody, in patients with mismatch repair-deficient tumors demonstrated its efficacy across all mismatch repair-deficient solid tumors[106,107] and led to the first tissue agnostic approval of a drug by the FDA in 2017.[108] The following year, a phase I/II basket study of larotrectinib in tumors with *TRK* fusions led to the second such FDA approval in 2018.[109] Basket trials are not always unmitigated successes, however. A study of vemurafenib in patients with advanced *BRAF*[V600] mutated malignancies (exclusive of melanoma) found an overall response rate of 42% of patients with NSCLC and 29% of those with anaplastic thyroid cancer,[110] leading to FDA approvals for dabrafenib in patients with V600E-mutated NSCLC[111] and anaplastic thyroid cancer.[112] However, few or no responses were observed in multiple other tumor types examined. Currently, multiple clinical trials are ongoing to evaluate the use of inhibitors of DNA damage repair in tumors with a variety of DNA damage repair-deficient mutations; preliminary results are encouraging[113] but still evolving.[114]

Umbrella trials have, to date, primarily served as exploratory signal-finding studies. They often operate using adaptive designs, wherein new arms may be added based on new evidence or removed based on lack of response, and patients may be assigned to a therapy based on an algorithm that uses evolving data to account for that patient's likelihood of response.[11] For example, the BATTLE studies assigned patients with advanced NSCLC to treatment arms based on molecular profiling of their tumors using real-time analyses of on-trial biopsies.[115,116]

The terms basket trial and umbrella trial are useful heuristics but may not adequately describe all large platform precision oncology trials.[117] A basket trial looking at patients whose tumors are DNA damage repair deficient, for example, examines a group of functionally similar molecular alterations. The ongoing NCI-MATCH (Molecular

Analysis for Therapy Choice) study uses on-study biopsies to assign patients with any histology to a broad range of therapies based on their tumor molecular alterations.[118] Although neither is a strict umbrella or basket trial, these hybrid platform studies enable the evaluation of multiple histologies and multiple mutations or other alterations.[12]

Master protocols present numerous challenges. They are time consuming, require significant coordination among multiple stakeholders, and can be costly.[13] Owing to their complexity, master protocols provide a difficult format for sponsors hoping to achieve registration and create significant work for regulatory officials and institutional review boards faced with numerous amendments.[11] They are rarely randomized, making it difficult to draw conclusions about the efficacy of an agent.[117] Varying statistical designs may limit the ability of investigators to draw definitive conclusions. For example, some basket studies are designed as a series of Simon 2-stage studies, treating each arm as a separate trial for statistical purposes and serving as a signal-finding study, whereas others allow aggregation of data from similar arms, which permits investigators to deem a therapy effective earlier.[119]

Despite these challenges, master protocols offer many opportunities for both patients and investigators. They enable patients with rare cancers to participate more readily in clinical trials and may lead to new therapeutic options. They efficiently group patients with multiple tumor types, are adaptable, and enable large collaborations.[11,13] They also can provide access to laboratories performing validated assessments of specific, treatment-defining molecular alterations in patients' tumors. Once established, the infrastructure for these trials can speed the screening of new therapeutic agents across a wide range of both common and understudied malignancies. However, platform trials are still in a relatively early stage of development.

SUMMARY

Rapid improvements in a variety of molecular characterization technologies over the past 2 decades have directly supported the development of new systemic cancer therapies that can be selected to target specific pharmacologic vulnerabilities in select patient populations across a wide range of human cancers. Molecular matching of drugs to specific targets for individual patients has substantively improved treatment for many hematological malignancies and solid tumors. Although this approach has become widespread only over the past 5 to 10 years, it has provided clinical benefits for many patients whose malignancies heretofore lacked effective therapy. Furthermore, in light of continuing improvements in our understanding of tumor biology and the tumor microenvironment, as well as remarkably efficient chemical biology and immunologic approaches now available for the development of therapeutics, further improvements in our ability to optimize cancer treatment based on the characteristics of an individual patient's tumor—the definition of precision oncology—are highly likely.

REFERENCES

1. Doroshow JH. Precision medicine in oncology. In: DeVita VT, Lawrence TS, Rosenberg SA, editors. Cancer: principles and practice of oncology. 11th edition. Philadelphia: Wolters Kluwer; 2019. p. 186–96.

2. Sparano JA, Gray RJ, Makower DF, et al. Adjuvant chemotherapy guided by a 21-Gene expression assay in breast cancer. N Engl J Med 2018;379:111–21.

3. Shaw AT, Felip E, Bauer TM, et al. Lorlatinib in non-small-cell lung cancer with ALK or ROS1 rearrangement: an international, multicentre, open-label, single-arm first-in-man phase 1 trial. Lancet Oncol 2017;18:1590–9.

4. Karapetis CS, Khambata-Ford S, Jonker DJ, et al. K-ras mutations and benefit from cetuximab in advanced colorectal cancer. N Engl J Med 2008;359: 1757–65.

5. Khorashad JS, Kelley TW, Szankasi P, et al. BCR-ABL1 compound mutations in tyrosine kinase inhibitor-resistant CML: frequency and clonal relationships. Blood 2013;121:489–98.

6. Editorial Board. Making precision oncology the standard of care. Lancet Oncol 2017;18:835.

7. Drilon A, Laetsch TW, Kummar S, et al. Efficacy of larotrectinib in TRK fusion-positive cancers in adults and children. N Engl J Med 2018;378:731–9.

8. DeVita VT, Chu E. A history of cancer chemotherapy. Cancer Res 2008;68: 8643–53.

9. Desmond-Hellmann S, Sawyers CL, Cox DR, et al. Toward precision medicine: building a knowledge network for biomedical research and a new taxonomy of disease. Washington, DC: National Academies Press; 2011.

10. Kummar S, Williams PM, Lih C-J, et al. Application of molecular profiling in clinical trials for advanced metastatic cancers. J Natl Cancer Inst 2015;107(4).

11. Cecchini M, Rubin EH, Blumenthal GM, et al. Challenges with novel clinical trial designs: master protocols. Clin Cancer Res 2019;25(7):2049–57.

12. Eckhardt SG, Lieu C. Is precision medicine an oxymoron? JAMA Oncol 2019; 5(2):142–3.

13. Woodcock J, LaVange LM. Master protocols to study multiple therapies, multiple diseases, or both. N Engl J Med 2017;377:62–70.

14. Slamon DJ, Clark GM, Wong SG, et al. Human breast cancer: correlation of relapse and survival with amplification of the HER-2/neu oncogene. Science 1987;235:177–82.

15. Slamon DJ, Godolphin W, Jones LA, et al. Studies of the HER-2/neu proto-oncogene in human breast and ovarian cancer. Science 1989;244:707–12.

16. Hudziak RM, Schlessinger J, Ullrich A. Increased expression of the putative growth factor receptor p185HER2 causes transformation and tumorigenesis of NIH 3T3 cells. Proc Natl Acad Sci U S A 1987;84:7159–63.

17. Di Fiore PP, Pierce JH, Kraus MH, et al. erbB-2 is a potent oncogene when over-expressed in NIH/3T3 cells. Science 1987;237:178–82.

18. Guy CT, Webster MA, Schaller M, et al. Expression of the neu protooncogene in the mammary epithelium of transgenic mice induces metastatic disease. Proc Natl Acad Sci U S A 1992;89:10578–82.

19. Carter P, Presta L, Gorman CM, et al. Humanization of an anti-p185HER2 antibody for human cancer therapy. Proc Natl Acad Sci U S A 1992;89:4285–9.

20. Baselga J. Clinical trials of Herceptin® (trastuzumab). Eur J Cancer 2001;37: 18–24.

21. Cobleigh MA, Vogel CL, Tripathy D, et al. Multinational study of the efficacy and safety of humanized anti-HER2 monoclonal antibody in women who have HER2-overexpressing metastatic breast cancer that has progressed after chemotherapy for metastatic disease. J Clin Oncol 1999;17:2639–48.

22. Roan S. Weapon in the war on cancer. Los Angeles Times 1998;S1.

23. Neergaard L. FDA looks at therapy for cancer; drug attacks gene linked to disease. Wash Post 1998;A10.

24. Slamon DJ, Leyland-Jones B, Shak S, et al. Use of chemotherapy plus a monoclonal antibody against HER2 for metastatic breast cancer that overexpresses HER2. N Engl J Med 2001;344:783–92.

25. Romond EH, Perez EA, Bryant J, et al. Trastuzumab plus adjuvant chemotherapy for operable HER2-positive breast cancer. N Engl J Med 2005;353:1673–84.

26. Smith I, Procter M, Gelber RD, et al. 2-year follow-up of trastuzumab after adjuvant chemotherapy in HER2-positive breast cancer: a randomised controlled trial. Lancet 2007;369:29–36.

27. Doroshow DB, LoRusso PM. Trastuzumab emtansine: determining its role in management of HER2+ breast cancer. Future Oncol 2018;14:589–602.

28. Gerratana L, Bonotto M, Bozza C, et al. Pertuzumab and breast cancer: another piece in the anti-HER2 puzzle. Expert Opin Biol Ther 2017;17:365–74.

29. Peres J. FDA OKs breakthrough leukemia pill. Chicago Tribune 2001. 1.26.

30. Druker BJ. Perspectives on the development of imatinib and the future of cancer research. Nat Med 2009;15:1149–52.

31. Druker BJ, Talpaz M, Resta DJ, et al. Efficacy and safety of a specific inhibitor of the BCR-ABL tyrosine kinase in chronic myeloid leukemia. N Engl J Med 2001;344:1031–7.

32. Cohen MH, Williams G, Johnson JR, et al. Approval summary for Imatinib Mesylate capsules in the treatment of chronic myelogenous leukemia. Clin Cancer Res 2002;8(5):935–42.

33. Goldman JM. Chronic myeloid leukemia: a historical perspective. Semin Hematol 2010;47:302–11.

34. Druker BJ. Translation of the Philadelphia chromosome into therapy for CML. Blood 2008;112:4808–17.

35. Nowell PC, Hungerford DA, National Academy of Sciences. A minute chromosome in human chronic granulocytic leukemia. Science 1960;132:1488–501.

36. Caspersson T, Gahrton G, Lindsten J, et al. Identification of the Philadelphia chromosome as a number 22 by quinacrine mustard fluorescence analysis. Exp Cell Res 1970;63:238–40.

37. O'Riordan ML, Robinson JA, Buckton KE, et al. Distinguishing between the chromosomes involved in Down's Syndrome (Trisomy 21) and chronic myeloid leukaemia (Ph 1) by fluorescence. Nature 1971;230:167.

38. Rowley JD. Letter: a new consistent chromosomal abnormality in chronic myelogenous leukaemia identified by quinacrine fluorescence and Giemsa staining. Nature 1973;243:290–3.

39. Davis RL, Konopka JB, Witte ON. Activation of the c-abl oncogene by viral transduction or chromosomal translocation generates altered c-abl proteins with similar in vitro kinase properties. Mol Cell Biol 1985;5:204–13.

40. Ben-Neriah Y, Daley GQ, Mes-Masson AM, et al. The chronic myelogenous leukemia-specific P210 protein is the product of the bcr/abl hybrid gene. Science 1986;233:212–4.

41. Daley GQ, Etten RV, Baltimore D. Induction of chronic myelogenous leukemia in mice by the P210bcr/abl gene of the Philadelphia chromosome. Science 1990;247:824–30.

42. Heisterkamp N, Jenster G, ten Hoeve J, et al. Acute leukaemia in bcr/abl transgenic mice. Nature 1990;344:251–3.

43. Bower H, Björkholm M, Dickman PW, et al. Life expectancy of patients With chronic myeloid leukemia approaches the life expectancy of the general population. J Clin Oncol 2016;34:2851–7.

44. Patel AB, Wilds BW, Deininger MW. Treating the chronic-phase chronic myeloid leukemia patient: which TKI, when to switch and when to stop? Expert Rev Hematol 2017;10:659–74.
45. Rusch V, Baselga J, Cordon-Cardo C, et al. Differential expression of the epidermal growth factor receptor and its ligands in primary non-small cell lung cancers and adjacent benign lung. Cancer Res 1993;53:2379–85.
46. Ranson M, Hammond LA, Ferry D, et al. ZD1839, a selective oral epidermal growth factor receptor-tyrosine kinase inhibitor, is well tolerated and active in patients with solid, malignant tumors: results of a phase I trial. J Clin Oncol 2002; 20:2240–50.
47. Herbst RS, Maddox A-M, Rothenberg ML, et al. Selective oral epidermal growth factor receptor tyrosine kinase inhibitor ZD1839 is generally well-tolerated and has activity in non-small-cell lung cancer and other solid tumors: results of a phase I trial. J Clin Oncol 2002;20:3815–25.
48. Baselga J, Rischin D, Ranson M, et al. Phase I safety, pharmacokinetic, and pharmacodynamic trial of ZD1839, a selective oral epidermal growth factor receptor tyrosine kinase inhibitor, in patients with five selected solid tumor types. J Clin Oncol 2002;20:4292–302.
49. Kris MG, Natale RB, Herbst RS, et al. Efficacy of gefitinib, an inhibitor of the epidermal growth factor receptor tyrosine kinase, in symptomatic patients with non-small cell lung cancer: a randomized trial. JAMA 2003;290:2149–58.
50. Fukuoka M, Yano S, Giaccone G, et al. Multi-institutional randomized phase II trial of gefitinib for previously treated patients with advanced non–small-cell lung cancer. J Clin Oncol 2003;21:2237–46.
51. Bailey R, Kris M, Wolf M, et al. O-242 Gefitinib ('Iressa', ZD1839) monotherapy for pretreated advanced non-small-cell lung cancer in IDEAL 1 and 2: tumor response is not clinically relevantly predictable from tumor EGFR membrane staining alone. Lung Cancer 2003;41:S71.
52. Cohen MH, Williams GA, Sridhara R, et al. United States Food and Drug Administration drug approval summary: gefitinib (ZD1839; Iressa) tablets. Clin Cancer Res 2004;10:1212–8.
53. Herbst RS, Giaccone G, Schiller JH, et al. Gefitinib in combination with paclitaxel and carboplatin in advanced non-small-cell lung cancer: a phase III trial–INTACT 2. J Clin Oncol 2004;22:785–94.
54. Giaccone G, Herbst RS, Manegold C, et al. Gefitinib in combination with gemcitabine and cisplatin in advanced non-small-cell lung cancer: a phase III trial–INTACT 1. J Clin Oncol 2004;22:777–84.
55. Jänne PA, Gurubhagavatula S, Yeap BY, et al. Outcomes of patients with advanced non-small cell lung cancer treated with gefitinib (ZD1839, "Iressa") on an expanded access study. Lung Cancer 2004;44:221–30.
56. Miller VA, Kris MG, Shah N, et al. Bronchioloalveolar pathologic subtype and smoking history predict sensitivity to gefitinib in advanced non–small-cell lung cancer. J Clin Oncol 2004;22:1103–9.
57. Pao W, Miller V, Zakowski M, et al. EGF receptor gene mutations are common in lung cancers from "never smokers" and are associated with sensitivity of tumors to gefitinib and erlotinib. Proc Natl Acad Sci U S A 2004;101:13306–11.
58. Paez JG, Jänne PA, Lee JC, et al. EGFR mutations in lung cancer: correlation with clinical response to gefitinib therapy. Science 2004;304:1497–500.
59. Lynch TJ, Bell DW, Sordella R, et al. Activating mutations in the epidermal growth factor receptor underlying responsiveness of non-small-cell lung cancer to gefitinib. N Engl J Med 2004;350:2129–39.

60. Oxnard GR, Arcila ME, Sima CS, et al. Acquired resistance to EGFR tyrosine kinase inhibitors in EGFR-mutant lung cancer: distinct natural history of patients with tumors harboring the T790M mutation. Clin Cancer Res 2011;17:1616–22.

61. Yu HA, Arcila ME, Rekhtman N, et al. Analysis of tumor specimens at the time of acquired resistance to EGFR-TKI therapy in 155 patients with EGFR-mutant lung cancers. Clin Cancer Res 2013;19:2240–7.

62. Yang JC-H, Ahn M-J, Kim D-W, et al. Osimertinib in pretreated T790M-positive advanced non-small-cell lung cancer: AURA study phase II extension component. J Clin Oncol 2017;35:1288–96.

63. Goss G, Tsai C-M, Shepherd FA, et al. Osimertinib for pretreated EGFR Thr790Met-positive advanced non-small-cell lung cancer (AURA2): a multi-centre, open-label, single-arm, phase 2 study. Lancet Oncol 2016;17:1643–52.

64. Mok TS, Wu Y-L, Ahn M-J, et al. Osimertinib or platinum-pemetrexed in EGFR T790M-positive lung cancer. N Engl J Med 2017;376:629–40.

65. Oxnard GR, Hu Y, Mileham KF, et al. Assessment of resistance mechanisms and clinical implications in patients with EGFR T790M-positive lung cancer and acquired resistance to osimertinib. JAMA Oncol 2018;4:1527–34.

66. Soria J-C, Ohe Y, Vansteenkiste J, et al. Osimertinib in untreated EGFR-mutated advanced non–small-cell lung cancer. N Engl J Med 2018;378:113–25.

67. Gainor JF, Shaw AT, Sequist LV, et al. EGFR mutations and ALK rearrangements are associated with low response rates to PD-1 pathway blockade in non-small cell lung cancer: a retrospective analysis. Clin Cancer Res 2016;22:4585–93.

68. Lisberg A, Cummings A, Goldman JW, et al. A phase II study of pembrolizumab in EGFR-mutant, PD-L1+, tyrosine kinase inhibitor naïve patients with advanced NSCLC. J Thorac Oncol 2018;13:1138–45.

69. Lee CK, Man J, Lord S, et al. Checkpoint inhibitors in metastatic EGFR-mutated non-small cell lung cancer-a meta-analysis. J Thorac Oncol 2017;12:403–7.

70. Ciardiello F, Tortora G. A novel approach in the treatment of cancer: targeting the epidermal growth factor receptor. Clin Cancer Res 2001;7:2958–70.

71. Cunningham D, Humblet Y, Siena S, et al. Cetuximab monotherapy and cetux-imab plus irinotecan in irinotecan-refractory metastatic colorectal cancer. N Engl J Med 2004;351:337–45.

72. Lièvre A, Bachet J-B, Le Corre D, et al. KRAS mutation status is predictive of response to cetuximab therapy in colorectal cancer. Cancer Res 2006;66:3992–5.

73. Di Fiore F, Blanchard F, Charbonnier F, et al. Clinical relevance of KRAS mutation detection in metastatic colorectal cancer treated by Cetuximab plus chemo-therapy. Br J Cancer 2007;96:1166–9.

74. Lièvre A, Bachet J-B, Boige V, et al. KRAS mutations as an independent prog-nostic factor in patients with advanced colorectal cancer treated with cetuxi-mab. J Clin Oncol 2008;26:374–9.

75. Allegra CJ, Rumble RB, Hamilton SR, et al. Extended RAS gene mutation testing in metastatic colorectal carcinoma to predict response to anti-epidermal growth factor receptor monoclonal antibody therapy: American Society of Clinical Oncology provisional clinical opinion update 2015. J Clin Oncol 2016;34:179–85.

76. Chapman PB, Hauschild A, Robert C, et al. Improved survival with vemurafenib in melanoma with BRAF V600E mutation. N Engl J Med 2011;364:2507–16.

77. Hauschild A, Grob J-J, Demidov LV, et al. Dabrafenib in BRAF-mutated metasta-tic melanoma: a multicentre, open-label, phase 3 randomised controlled trial. Lancet 2012;380:358–65.

78. Paraiso KHT, Fedorenko IV, Cantini LP, et al. Recovery of phospho-ERK activity allows melanoma cells to escape from BRAF inhibitor therapy. Br J Cancer 2010; 102:1724–30.

79. Sosman JA, Kim KB, Schuchter L, et al. Survival in BRAF V600–mutant advanced melanoma treated with vemurafenib. N Engl J Med 2012;366:707–14.

80. Sosman JA, Pavlick AC, Schuchter LM, et al. Analysis of molecular mechanisms of response and resistance to vemurafenib (vem) in BRAFV600E melanoma. J Clin Oncol 2012;30(15_suppl):8503.

81. Long GV, Stroyakovskiy D, Gogas H, et al. Combined BRAF and MEK inhibition versus BRAF inhibition alone in melanoma. N Engl J Med 2014;371:1877–88.

82. Long GV, Stroyakovskiy D, Gogas H, et al. Dabrafenib and trametinib versus dabrafenib and placebo for Val600 BRAF-mutant melanoma: a multicentre, double-blind, phase 3 randomised controlled trial. Lancet 2015;386:444–51.

83. Long GV, Flaherty KT, Stroyakovskiy D, et al. Dabrafenib plus trametinib versus dabrafenib monotherapy in patients with metastatic BRAF V600E/K-mutant melanoma: long-term survival and safety analysis of a phase 3 study. Ann Oncol 2017;28:1631–9.

84. Robert C, Karaszewska B, Schachter J, et al. Improved overall survival in melanoma with combined dabrafenib and trametinib. N Engl J Med 2015;372:30–9.

85. Holbeck SL, Camalier R, Crowell JA, et al. The National Cancer Institute ALMANAC: a comprehensive screening resource for the detection of anticancer drug pairs with enhanced therapeutic activity. Cancer Res 2017;77:3564–76.

86. Wolff AC, Hammond MEH, Allison KH, et al. HER2 testing in breast cancer: American Society of Clinical Oncology/College of American Pathologists clinical practice guideline focused update summary. J Oncol Pract 2018;14:437–41.

87. Roychowdhury S, Iyer MK, Robinson DR, et al. Personalized oncology through integrative high-throughput sequencing: a pilot study. Sci Transl Med 2011;3: 111ra121.

88. Garraway LA, Lander ES. Lessons from the cancer genome. Cell 2013;153: 17–37.

89. CMS finalizes coverage of Next Generation Sequencing tests, ensuring enhanced access for cancer patients | CMS. Available at: https://www.cms.gov/newsroom/press-releases/cms-finalizes-coverage-next-generation-sequencing-tests-ensuring-enhanced-access-cancer-patients. Accessed April 14, 2019.

90. Jones S, Anagnostou V, Lytle K, et al. Personalized genomic analyses for cancer mutation discovery and interpretation. Sci Transl Med 2015;7:283ra53.

91. Yap TA, Sandhu SK, Workman P, et al. Envisioning the future of early anticancer drug development. Nat Rev Cancer 2010;10:514–23.

92. Gainor JF, Longo DL, Chabner BA. Pharmacodynamic biomarkers: falling short of the mark? Clin Cancer Res 2014;20:2587–94.

93. Goldberg SB, Patel AA. Monitoring immunotherapy outcomes with circulating tumor DNA. Immunotherapy 2018;10:1023–5.

94. Tannock IF, Hickman JA. Limits to personalized cancer medicine. N Engl J Med 2016;375:1289–94.

95. Hyman DM, Taylor BS, Baselga J. Implementing genome-driven oncology. Cell 2017;168:584–99.

96. McGranahan N, Swanton C. Clonal heterogeneity and tumor evolution: past, present, and the future. Cell 2017;168:613–28.

97. Rübben A, Araujo A. Cancer heterogeneity: converting a limitation into a source of biologic information. J Transl Med 2017;15:190.

98. Redig AJ, Jänne PA. Basket trials and the evolution of clinical trial design in an era of genomic medicine. J Clin Oncol 2015;33(9):975–7.
99. Dienstmann R, Rodon J, Tabernero J. Optimal design of trials to demonstrate the utility of genomically-guided therapy: putting precision cancer medicine to the test. Mol Oncol 2015;9:940–50.
100. André F, Bachelot T, Commo F, et al. Comparative genomic hybridisation array and DNA sequencing to direct treatment of metastatic breast cancer: a multicentre, prospective trial (SAFIR01/UNICANCER). Lancet Oncol 2014;15: 267–74.
101. Tsimberidou A-M, Iskander NG, Hong DS, et al. Personalized medicine in a phase I clinical trials program: the MD Anderson Cancer Center initiative. Clin Cancer Res 2012;18:6373–83.
102. Kris MG, Johnson BE, Berry LD, et al. Using multiplexed assays of oncogenic drivers in lung cancers to select targeted drugs. JAMA 2014;311:1998–2006.
103. Sohal DPS, Rini BI, Khorana AA, et al. Prospective clinical study of precision oncology in solid tumors. J Natl Cancer Inst 2016;108(3) [pii:djv332].
104. Bedard PL, Oza A, Clarke B, et al. Abstract PR03: molecular profiling of advanced solid tumors at Princess Margaret Cancer Centre and patient outcomes with genotype-matched clinical trials. Clin Cancer Res 2016; 22(1 Supplement):PR03.
105. Le Tourneau C, Delord J-P, Gonçalves A, et al. Molecularly targeted therapy based on tumour molecular profiling versus conventional therapy for advanced cancer (SHIVA): a multicentre, open-label, proof-of-concept, randomised, controlled phase 2 trial. Lancet Oncol 2015;16:1324–34.
106. Le DT, Uram JN, Wang H, et al. PD-1 blockade in tumors with mismatch-repair deficiency. N Engl J Med 2015;372:2509–20.
107. Le DT, Durham JN, Smith KN, et al. Mismatch repair deficiency predicts response of solid tumors to PD-1 blockade. Science 2017;357:409–13.
108. Approved Drugs - FDA grants accelerated approval to pembrolizumab for first tissue/site agnostic indication. Available at: https://www.fda.gov/drugs/informationondrugs/approveddrugs/ucm560040.htm. Accessed April 10, 2019.
109. Approved Drugs - FDA approves larotrectinib for solid tumors with NTRK gene fusions. Available at: https://www.fda.gov/drugs/informationondrugs/approveddrugs/ucm626720.htm. Accessed April 10, 2019.
110. Hyman DM, Puzanov I, Subbiah V, et al. Vemurafenib in multiple nonmelanoma cancers with BRAF V600 mutations. N Engl J Med 2015;373:726–36.
111. Approved Drugs - FDA grants regular approval to dabrafenib and trametinib combination for metastatic NSCLC with BRAF V600E mutation. Available at: https://www.fda.gov/drugs/informationondrugs/approveddrugs/ucm564331.htm. Accessed April 10, 2019.
112. Approved Drugs - FDA approves dabrafenib plus trametinib for anaplastic thyroid cancer with BRAF V600E mutation. Available at: https://www.fda.gov/drugs/informationondrugs/approveddrugs/ucm606708.htm. Accessed April 15, 2019.
113. Mateo J, Carreira S, Sandhu S, et al. DNA-repair defects and olaparib in metastatic prostate cancer. N Engl J Med 2015;373:1697–708.
114. Gruber JJ, Afghahi A, Hatton A, et al. Talazoparib beyond BRCA: a phase II trial of talazoparib monotherapy in BRCA1 and BRCA2 wild-type patients with advanced HER2-negative breast cancer or other solid tumors with a mutation in homologous recombination (HR) pathway genes. J Clin Oncol 2019; 37(suppl). abstr 3006.

115. Kim ES, Herbst RS, Wistuba II, et al. The BATTLE trial: personalizing therapy for lung cancer. Cancer Discov 2011;1:44–53.
116. Papadimitrakopoulou V, Lee JJ, Wistuba II, et al. The BATTLE-2 study: a biomarker-integrated targeted therapy study in previously treated patients with advanced non-small-cell lung cancer. J Clin Oncol 2016;34:3638–47.
117. Janiaud P, Serghiou S, Ioannidis JPA. New clinical trial designs in the era of precision medicine: an overview of definitions, strengths, weaknesses, and current use in oncology. Cancer Treat Rev 2019;73:20–30.
118. Conley BA, Doroshow JH. Molecular analysis for therapy choice: NCI MATCH. Semin Oncol 2014;41:297–9.
119. Cunanan KM, Gonen M, Shen R, et al. Basket trials in oncology: a trade-off between complexity and efficiency. J Clin Oncol 2017;35:271–3.

Precision Medicine and Targeted Therapies in Breast Cancer

Ian Greenwalt, MD[a], Norah Zaza, BA[b], Shibandri Das, MD[a],
Benjamin D. Li, MD, MBA[c],*

KEYWORDS

- Breast cancer • Precision medicine • Targeted therapy • Endocrine therapy • HER2
- Multigene array • Genomics • Radiomics

KEY POINTS

- Discuss the current state of breast cancer care including endocrine therapy, anti-HER2 therapy and chemotherapy.
- Discuss the current state of precision medicine including molecular subtyping and gene expression profiles.
- Discuss the role of genomics and radiomics in precision medicine and breast cancer care.

INTRODUCTION

Progress made in our understanding of genomics, proteomics, and cancer biology has led to a deeper appreciation for the complexity and variability in a tumor's genotypic and phenotypic expression, and the complex malignant transformation known as cancer. Consequently, cancer treatment has also begun to evolve toward a more individualized, precise and targeted approach for each patient and the specific cancer that has been diagnosed, based on the complexity of the molecular profile of the tumor and the patient. This has marked the beginning of the era toward precision medicine and targeted therapeutics.

The evolution in breast cancer therapy serves as a prime example for this nascent journey. In the following article, a review of the history of targeted therapy in breast cancer, an update on its current state, and the role precision medicine has played

Disclosure Statement: The authors have nothing to disclose.
[a] University Hospitals Cleveland Medical Center, MetroHealth Hospitals, Louis Stokes Veterans Administration Hospital, Case Western Reserve University, Cleveland, OH, USA; [b] Case Western Reserve University, Cleveland, OH, USA; [c] MetroHealth System, Case Western Reserve University, Cancer Care Pavilion, Suite C2100, 2500 MetroHealth Drive, Cleveland, OH 44109-1998, USA
* Corresponding author.
E-mail address: bli@metrohealth.org

in breast cancer care are highlighted. The overarching goal is to provide an overview of how precision medicine has impacted breast cancer management as an example of the early progress made in precision medicine and targeted therapy in cancer care.

TARGETED THERAPIES IN BREAST CANCER
Endocrine Therapy

Tamoxifen is the earliest and best studied example of targeted therapy in our anti-cancer armamentarium. As a selective estrogen receptor modulator that can competitively bind to the estrogen receptor (ER) on cell surfaces of breast cancer cells, tamoxifen has been shown to improve disease-free survival in premenopausal and postmenopausal women with breast cancer since the 1970s.[1,2] In postmenopausal women, response rates of the cancer were on the order of 50% to 70% for those with ER-positive ± progesterone receptor (PR)-positive tumors. In contrast, there is a less than 10% response rate for those patients with ER-negative/PR-negative tumors. In the adjuvant setting, pooling the results of multiple clinical trials, the Early Breast Cancer Trialists' Collaborative Group (EBCTCG) reported the impact of tamoxifen on patients with ER-positive breast cancer. These findings showed an improvement in 10-year survival by 10.9% for node-positive (61.4% vs 50.5% survival, $P<.00001$) and 5.6% for node-negative (78.9% vs 73.3% survival, $P<.00001$) breast cancer.[3] In male breast cancer, in which the disease is rare but has been found to be more likely positive for ERs, tamoxifen has an overall response rate of 50% in unselected male patients but increases to 71% in patients with ER-positive tumors. Finally, the EBCTCG also reported that adjuvant tamoxifen therapy reduced the risk of development of contralateral breast cancer by 39% compared with no adjuvant therapy.[2]

Aromatase inhibitors (AI) offered the next development in targeting hormone receptor–positive breast cancers. Aromatase catalyzes the conversion of androgens to estrogens and can be used to decrease levels of circulating estrogen, specifically in postmenopausal women.[1,4] The 2 categories of AI are Type 1 steroidals and Type II nonsteroidals. Type I steroidals include formestane and exemestane. These bind competitively to aromatase enzyme. Type II nonsteroidals, such as anastrozole and letrozole, bind reversibly to aromatase and require continued drug presence in the body for sustained inhibition.

Today, the 3 most commonly used and orally available agents are emestane, anastrozole, and letrozole. There have been 2 large randomized phase 3 trials: (1) the North American trial and (2) TARGET trial. These 2 trials compared tamoxifen versus AI efficacy in reducing cancer recurrence. In TARGET, anastrozole 1 mg/d orally showed equivalence with comparison to tamoxifen 20 mg/d orally in terms of median time to disease progression and clinical benefit rate. In the North American trial, the results showed a significant improvement in median time to disease progression of 11.1 months with anastrozole, compared with 5.6 months with tamoxifen. In addition, in a phase 3 head-to-head trial, Mouridsen and colleagues[5] demonstrated that letrozole achieved better results when compared with tamoxifen alone. Women treated with letrozole had a 3-month improvement in time to progression, as well as longer time to chemotherapy when compared with tamoxifen.[4]

Human Epidermal Growth Factor Receptor 2 Therapy

The discovery of trastuzumab, a monoclonal antibody (MAB) that inhibits the extracellular domain of the human epidermal growth factor receptor 2 (HER2) receptor, is seen as the beginning of a new era in targeted therapy for breast cancer.[1] HER2 can homodimerize or heterodimerize, both of which lead to activation of PI3K/AKT pathways.

The addition of trastuzumab, either concurrently or sequentially, to chemotherapy regimens improves both overall survival (OS) and disease-free progression (DFS) (hazard ratio [HR] 0.66; 95% confidence interval [CI] 0.57–0.77, P<.00001; and HR 0.60; 95% CI 0.50–0.71, P<.00001, respectively).[6] Pertuzumab is another MAB that acts on HER2. It inhibits the heterodimerization domain and in tumor models, trastuzumab and pertuzumab have been found to have synergistic antitumor activity. This was subsequently confirmed in the CLEOPATRA trial. In this study, patients with HER2-positive, metastatic disease with no prior treatment were randomly assigned to trastuzumab and docetaxel, plus either pertuzumab or placebo. There was an increase in progression-free survival (PFS) of 6 months and OS of 16 months when pertuzumab was added to trastuzumab.[7]

MAB targeting of HER2 also has made inroads in the adjuvant management of breast cancer. Pertuzumab was evaluated as an addition to adjuvant trastuzumab and chemotherapy in patients with HER2-positive, nonmetastatic, breast cancer after surgical resection. The adjuvant therapy regimen was initiated within 8 weeks of surgery. Patients were assigned to standard chemotherapy and trastuzumab plus pertuzumab or standard chemotherapy and trastuzumab plus placebo for 1 year. Pertuzumab and trastuzumab with chemotherapy led to a 94.1% rate of DFS. It was 93.2% in the placebo group. In the cohort of patients with node-positive disease, the 3-year rate of invasive DFS was 92.0% in the pertuzumab group compared with 90.2% in the placebo group (HR for invasive-disease event, 0.77; 95% CI 0.62–0.96; P = .02).[8]

Another role for anti-HER2 therapies in the adjuvant setting is the novel combination of trastuzumab with a cytotoxic chemotherapeutic agent, emtansine (TDM1). This conjugate works by inhibiting HER2 signaling (via trastuzumab) and also prevents microtubule function (via DM1). A study investigated the risk of recurrence of invasive breast cancer in those with residual invasive disease treated with TDM1 and trastuzumab compared with trastuzumab alone in the adjuvant setting. The study group was made up of patients with HER2-positive, nonmetastatic breast cancer treated with neoadjuvant therapy with residual disease found on surgical pathology. The group then received the 2 adjuvant regimens. Comparative results demonstrated that those treated with adjuvant TDM1 had a 50% lower risk of recurrence or death than those with trastuzumab alone.[9]

RECENT DEVELOPMENTS IN TARGETED THERAPY INVOLVING OTHER MOLECULAR PATHWAYS
Mammalian Target of Rapamycin Pathway Inhibitors

In studying patients with hormone receptor–positive, advanced stage breast cancer who developed resistance to endocrine therapies, it was discovered that their tumors had upregulation of the mammalian target of rapamycin (mTOR) kinase pathway.[1] Based on this discovery, it was later found that a combination of mTOR inhibition along with anti-endocrine therapies, had resulted in improved survival in patients with breast cancer. As Baselga and colleagues[10] demonstrated, the use of mTOR inhibitors with AIs created a synergistic effect that can cease proliferation and induce apoptosis of hormone receptor–positive tumors in patients with advanced disease. Through this combination of everolimus with AI, there was improved PFS from 2.8 to 6.9 months when compared with AI alone (HR 0.43; 95% CI 0.35–0.54; P<.001).

This therapeutic strategy was then applied to the management of disease initially refractory to endocrine therapies. In patients with unfavorable response to first-line AI agents, such as letrozole or anastrozole, combining exemestane with everolimus provided improved PFS. This was supported by the results of the phase 2, randomized controlled trial BOLERO-6 study of everolimus plus exemestane versus everolimus alone (PFS HR of 0.74, 90% CI 0.57–0.97).[11]

Inhibition of the mTOR pathway has further applications in delaying or preventing resistance to endocrine therapies. Royce and colleagues[12] postulated that dual inhibition targeting mTOR and hormone receptor–positive tumors could delay or prevent endocrine resistance by weeding out hormone independent cell lines with early dual therapy. This multicenter, phase 2 clinical trial demonstrated PFS of 22 months (95% CI 18.1–25.1 months) with the use of everolimus and letrozole compared with letrozole alone. Before this study, PFS was typically 9.0 to 9.4 months.

Cyclin Dependent Kinase 4 and 6 Pathway Inhibitors

Another targeted therapy strategy involves the Cyclin Dependent Kinase 4 and 6 (CDK 4/6) pathway. CDK 4/6 plays a central role in the phosphorylation of the Rb protein, which allows the progression of G1 to S phase in the cell cycle.[1] Upregulating the phosphorylation of the Rb protein has been demonstrated in hormone-resistant breast cancer cells. Medications such as ribociclib, abemaciclib, and palbociclib are small molecules that can inhibit the CDK 4/6 pathway, shutting down the cell cycle, and leading to apoptosis of cancer cells. Similar to the combination of mTOR inhibitors and AI, the dual use of CDK 4/6 inhibitors with AI has a synergistic effect on hormone receptor–positive breast cancers. There has been a demonstrable improvement in PFS with the use of palbociclib and letrozole compared with letrozole alone in patients with hormone receptor–positive, HER2-negative, advanced stage breast cancer. Finn and colleagues[13] showed this in PALOMA-1/TRIO-18 with a PFS of 20.2 months in the palbociclib and letrozole arm compared with PFS of 10.2 months in the letrozole group.

There also appears to be an application for CDK 4/6 inhibition in breast cancers that have displayed endocrine resistance. In patients with hormone receptor–positive, HER2-negative breast cancer with advanced disease that had demonstrated previous resistance to endocrine therapies, Sledge and colleagues[14] reported that the combined use of abemaciclib with fulvestrant resulted in a PFS of 16.4 months versus 9.3 months with fulvestrant alone (HR 0.553; 95% CI 0.449–0.681). There was also tumor size reduction with a mean decrease in tumor size of 62.5% for the abemaciclib and fulvestrant arm compared with 32.8% for the control arm.

Poly ADP-Ribose Polymerase Inhibitors

Poly ADP-Ribose Polymerase (PARP) is one of the means by which cells attempt to maintain genomic integrity. In the presence of single-strand DNA breaks, PARP is activated and acts as both a signal and a platform for DNA repair proteins.[15] Otherwise, the damage may result in cell death. BRCA1 and BRCA2 gene products are proteins important in the repair of double-strand DNA breaks. BRCA gene mutations can lead to errors in DNA repair that can eventually result in breast cancer formation in normal breast cells. When subjected to enough damage in DNA and where the mechanisms of repair are severely compromised, cell death, even among cancer cells, can occur.

PARP inhibitors block the repair of single-strand DNA breaks. If these unrepaired nicks persist during DNA replication, double-strand breaks can form. In breast cancer with BRCA mutations, these double breaks cannot be efficiently repaired. As a result, the breast cancer cells die. Normal breast cells without BRCA mutation still have their repair mechanism intact. Thus, they can survive the inhibition of PARP.

PARP inhibitors, such as olaparib and talazoparib, have been shown to improve the outcomes for patients with BRCA-positive breast cancer.[15] Robson and colleagues[16] and Litton and colleagues[17] illustrated the efficacy of PARP inhibitors in patients with metastatic BRCA-positive breast cancer by achieving improved PFS as well as decreased risk of disease progression, decreased risk of death, and delay in time to clinical deterioration. Specifically, the median PFS for the olaparib group was 2.8 months longer than the standard chemotherapy group (HR for disease progression or death of 0.58; 95% CI 0.43–0.80; $P<.001$).

THE ROLE OF PRECISION MEDICINE IN DETERMINING TREATMENT

In 2011, the National Research Council released a consensus study report with the proposal to redefine disease based on molecular and environmental determinants, rather than using traditional signs, symptoms, and traditional histology.[18] The potential for harnessing big data networks and expanding molecular signatures to redefine disease, tailoring a personalized treatment regimen based on an individual's unique molecular profile along with other determinants, can result in far more efficacious treatments, and with far fewer treatment-related complications. This very concept is being tested out in a nascent manner in cancer therapy, more specifically, in our approach to breast cancer treatment.

Molecular Subtyping and Treatment Decision

In the previous section, examples of targeted agents in response to actionable mutations in critical molecular pathways were exploited to inhibit or kill tumor cells. Molecular subtyping of cancer also can aid in the decision of whether standard systemic therapy, such as standard cytotoxic chemotherapy, should be part of adjuvant therapy in breast cancer. Although cytotoxic chemotherapy has demonstrated benefits in DFS and OS, these benefits are not universal in the population treated; nor are the degree and susceptibility for adverse events experienced equally. The tumor's biology, the patient's constitution, and the clinical setting all play a role in maximizing the benefits of treatment, and in minimizing the potential for morbid or toxic outcomes. We are just beginning to appreciate and to stratify some of these determinants.

In breast cancer, examples of some such early developments and applications are in the multigene arrays now quite routinely applied to tumor specimens. These include the 3 most commonly used multigene arrays in clinical use today: Oncotype DX, MammaPrint, and PAM50 (Predication Analysis of Microarrays) (**Table 1**). They each

Table 1
Common breast cancer multigene arrays

Test	Composition	Type of Cancer	Application
Oncotype DX	21-gene assay	ER/PR+, node−	Classify early-stage breast cancers into low, intermediate, and high risk of recurrence within 10 y. Help guide use of chemotherapy and radiation.
MammaPrint	70-gene assay	ER/PR+ or ER/PR−	Applied to patient with intermediate risk of recurrence. Stratifies patients into good or poor prognostic risk of metastatic disease.
PAM50	50-gene assay	ER/PR+, node+	Predicts likelihood of recurrence within 10 y.

Abbreviations: ER/PR, estrogen receptor/progesterone receptor, PAM50, Predication Analysis of Microarrays.

represent the next step in individualizing the decision making for chemotherapy for patients with breast cancer.

In Oncotype DX, this multigene array is derived from 21 genes originally studied in patients with ER-positive, lymph node–negative cancers who were treated with tamoxifen. These findings have been extrapolated to patients with early-stage breast cancer and used as a tool to classify patients as low, intermediate, or high risk for recurrence. Based on the risk stratification for recurrence, Oncotype DX results help guide chemotherapy decisions for these patients.[19] This 21-gene array also has been shown to be predictive for locoregional recurrence. As such, Oncotype DX also has a role to play in the selection for adjuvant radiation therapy.

MammaPrint is another multigene array, based on the analysis of 70 genes known to influence tumor growth, signaling, replication, and cell death. MammaPrint is often applied to patients with intermediate risk for recurrent disease. The assay stratifies patients into those with a good versus poor prognostic signature for distant metastasis. Its applicability includes those patients with HER2-positive and node-positive breast cancer. This subset of patients is not usually amenable to Oncotype DX testing alone. MammaPrint is used to aid in the selection of chemotherapies and in providing patients and their treating physicians with additional prognostic information.[19]

Last, PAM50 is an analytical tool designed to classify intrinsic molecular subtyping. The assay estimates a risk for recurrence score to better characterize, classify, and treat patients with early ER-positive, HER2-negative breast cancer. The risk profiling was based on an initial cohort of postmenopausal patients with early ER-positive, HER2-negative tumors, treated with neoadjuvant endocrine therapy, and their related response to neoadjuvant or adjuvant chemotherapy. PAM50 is a microarray of 50 genes.[19]

Gene Expression Profile and Breast Cancer

It can be argued that the era of molecular characterization to determine treatment for breast cancer began when the gene expression profiles of several hundred complementary DNA clones extracted from 78 breast carcinomas were studied in attempt to create a new classification of breast cancer based on the molecular signature obtained.[20] The intent is that a better understanding of a tumor's molecular profile can lead to improved abilities to determine prognosis and enhanced precision in treatment decisions. Since the introduction of breast cancer intrinsic subtype classification, the ability to better predict risk for recurrence, the option to select targeted therapy based on molecular profiling, and a greater degree of precision in therapeutic decision making has resulted in improved clinical outcomes.[21]

Tumor response to treatment is not determined by traditional anatomic prognostic factors, such as tumor size and nodal status. Rather, intrinsic molecular characteristics of each individual tumor, as captured by its array of gene expression, are more informative in predicting treatment response and clinical outcomes. Further developments in the classification of breast cancer based on expression profile will gain in utility and function, as expression profile through microarray and high-throughput analysis become more feasible and prevalent.

Currently, breast tumors can be grouped into 4 molecular subtypes, based on 4 well-established molecular markers. These include hormone receptor ER and PR positivity, HER2 receptor status, and the proliferation index of Ki67. The 4 subtypes identified make up most breast cancers. They are luminal A, luminal B, HER2 overexpression, and basal-like tumors (**Table 2**). Luminal A is described as ER positive with/without PR positivity, HER2-negative, and with less than 14% presence of Ki67. Luminal B is divided into HER2-positive and negative groups, with ER-positive and/or

Table 2
Breast cancer subtypes

Subtype	Molecular Characteristics	Treatment	Response
Luminal A (most common)	ER+, +/− PR, HER2-negative, <14% Ki67	Endocrine therapy	Excellent prognosis. Responds well to Endocrine therapy, not well to chemotherapy.
Luminal B	ER+, +/− PR HER2-positive/negative >14% Ki67	Endocrine and chemotherapy	Worse prognosis. More aggressive than luminal A.
HER2 overexpression	ER and PR-negative HER2-positive, any amount Ki67	Chemotherapy and anti-HER2 therapy	Poor prognosis vs luminal subtypes.
Basal-like	Triple negative, any amount Ki67	Chemotherapy	Very poor prognosis.

Abbreviations: ER, estrogen receptor; HER2, human epidermal growth factor receptor 2; PR, progesterone receptor.

PR-positive hormone status, and a greater than 14% presence of Ki67. The HER2 overexpression tumors are ER and PR negative, HER2 positive, and with any amount of Ki67. Finally, the basal-like subtype has triple negative receptors, with a varying amount of Ki67 presence.[19,20]

Understanding the subtypes and the mutations associated with each provides insight on the prognosis of each subtype, as well as helps in therapeutic decision making. Luminal A is the most common subtype. As an ER-positive and/or PR-positive tumor, it has an excellent prognosis, likely because of the associated low proliferative index score, and a well-differentiated cancer by histologic examination. It responds well to hormone therapy, but poorly to chemotherapy. As such, patients with luminal A breast cancer do well with endocrine therapy and may forego adjuvant chemotherapy.[21]

Luminal B subtype has a higher index of proliferation. It is also associated with a worse prognosis, with a disease course that is significantly more aggressive than luminal A breast cancer. It is more often associated with poorly differentiated histology and a higher frequency for bone metastases. A combined therapeutic strategy of endocrine therapy with chemotherapy is often used to optimize outcomes.[21]

HER2 overexpression subtype has a very high proliferative index and is most often poorly differentiated by histology. Also, in 40% to 80% of the patients, it is associated with the p53 mutation. It has a poor prognosis and a lower survival rate than both luminal subtypes. They are sensitive to anthracycline and taxane-based neoadjuvant chemotherapy though, with a significantly higher pathologic complete response than luminal tumors. However, incomplete tumor eradication by therapy results in early relapse. As these tumors are HER2 positive, patients are candidates for and are responsive to anti-HER2 targeted therapy.[21]

The basal-like subtype is composed of triple negative breast cancer (TNBC). Receptor status of these tumors are ER, PR, and HER2 negative. However, not all TNBCs belong to the basal-like subtype. This subtype of tumors resembles the expression profile of basal epithelial cells in other organs. The cancer tends toward being poorly differentiated, a high proliferative index, mitotic index, and associated with p53 mutations.[22] The patients with this subtype of breast cancer tend to have experienced menarche at a younger age, and being multiparous is not protective like in the luminal subtype. The tumor at presentation tends to be larger, grows more rapidly, and when metastatic, is less likely to be associated with initial node-positive disease. Disseminated disease also tends toward visceral organs.

Overall, the prognosis for this subtype of breast cancer is very poor. Although this subtype is associated with low ER, PR, and HER2 expression, it has high expression for basal markers, such as cytokeratin markers. As basal-like subtype of breast cancer lacks these receptors, it lacks response to the currently available targeted therapy designed for these receptors. Therefore, chemotherapy is the only option in the current treatment armamentarium. Both paclitaxel and doxorubicin-containing neoadjuvant chemotherapies have been shown to produce the best pathologic response among basal-like subtypes.[23]

In general, the luminal subtypes do not appear to be as sensitive to neoadjuvant chemotherapy as the more aggressive subtypes.[23] Caudle and colleagues[24] demonstrated that luminal A and B tumors had significantly lower rates of pathologic complete response (9% and 18%, respectively) compared with patients with HER2 overexpression and basal-like tumors (36% and 38%, respectively).[23] In light of this, preoperative chemotherapy should be strongly considered before surgical intervention for the nonluminal subtypes.

The progression to the use of intrinsic subtype classification in breast cancer in the treatment decision is fundamentally different from the use of tumor markers as prognosticators for cancer outcomes. Using individual prognostic markers as predictors for cancer outcomes do not capture the molecular complexity intrinsic to breast cancer tumors. Gene expression profile using microarray analysis will eventually be able to capture a more precise and comprehensive characterization of the molecular signature of a complex tumor specimen at diagnosis, and as it progresses in its disease course. This allows for adjustment of the therapeutic strategy to a more precise approach to targeted therapy, acting at a specific defective pathway. One such ongoing proof-of-concept trial of matching a defect in a molecular pathway with a specific potential targeted therapy is the recently completed MATCH trial, sponsored by the ECOG-ACRIN group.[25]

Radiomics

Precision medicine to better individualize treatment based on a patient and the tumor's characteristics has applications in radiation therapy. Adjuvant and therapeutic application of radiotherapy is a standard model in breast cancer treatment. At present, individualization of radiotherapy for a patient's tumor involve primarily anatomic precision and imaging features.[26]

Radiomics is a developing science in the extraction of many features from radiographic images using data-characterization algorithms to potentially uncover disease characteristics. With regard to breast cancer, the study of radiomics attempts to correlate a tumor's radiographic features with its intrinsic subtype and molecular profile with the end goal of using this information to help identify clinical outcomes.[26] Specific examples can be seen in the work of Fan and colleagues[27] who reported that with MRI, there is less tumor heterogeneity in less aggressive cancers, like the luminal A subtype. In addition, HER2 overexpression subtype was found to have the highest enhancement value on MRI.

Advancement in breast ultrasound and digital mammography technology also may be used to determine certain biologic characteristics of breast cancer, as well as their Ki67 status. With ultrasound, low-grade tumors tend to have more irregular shapes and are hyperechoic. In contrast, high-grade tumors tend to have a regular shape and are more hypoechoic.[26] Ma and colleagues[28] used 39 features of digital mammography to differentiate subtypes of breast cancer, finding that each tumor subtype was significantly associated with 4 of these features: roundness, concavity, gray mean, and correlation.[26]

Radiomics also plays a role in determining recurrence risk. Drukker and colleagues[29] reported that certain MRI features correlate with recurrent breast cancer. The MRI feature most closely associated with earlier cancer recurrence was the Most Enhancing Tumor Volume (METV). The METV obtained before and after the first cycle of neoadjuvant chemotherapy was reliable in predicting earlier cancer recurrence.

Further application of precision medicine is found at the junction of genomics and radiomics. Investigators have established a genome-adjusted radiation dose (GARD) using gene-expression–based radiation-sensitivity index and a linear quadratic model that describes biological response to radiation.[30] This model is an attempt to facilitate adjustment of radiotherapy dose and predict the effect of radiation therapy. Although this model was tested in several cancers, the breast cancer cohort was further studied to establish a GARD threshold that was associated with better clinical outcomes.[30] Similarly, the MATCH trial mentioned earlier should provide further insight into radiomics, as part of the study design was to examine the potential utility of high-throughput radiologic data in the characterization of tumors and its response to treatment.[25]

Precision Medicine in Breast Surgery

Surgical options in the treatment of breast cancer can be generally simplified into (1) total mastectomy versus partial mastectomy (PM), and (2) nodal staging by sentinel node biopsy (SLN) versus a complete axillary node dissection. The choice of surgery depends on the stage of the breast cancer at presentation, the overall health of the patient, and each patient's preference. That being said, the most commonly performed surgical treatment is PM plus SLN, known commonly as breast conservation surgery (BCS). This is because with the prevalence of the breast cancer screening program, the disease is most commonly diagnosed at a clinically node-negative stage, with a tumor smaller than 5 cm.

Recent studies have begun to investigate clinical outcomes of the different breast cancer subtypes to the various surgical options. Each of the 4 subtypes (luminal A, luminal B, HER2 overexpression, and basal-like) appear to hold different nuances in their response to BCS and radiation therapy. Although all 4 subtypes had a less than 10% recurrence rate at 5 years following BCS, luminal A subtype had a particularly low recurrence rate of 0.8% (luminal B 1.5%, HER2 overexpression 8.4%, basal-like 7.1%).[31] The rate of positive nodes after SLN also varies based on subtype. The highest frequencies of positive SLN were 44.9% and 50.0% among luminal B and HER2 overexpression subtypes, respectively ($P = .0003$).[32] Further improvements in subtyping and more precision in correlation of outcome can potentially lead to the elimination of adjuvant radiation therapy for a specific subtype, or to eliminate the need to perform surgical axillary staging in another subtype.

Radiomics also can potentially impact surgical treatment. As supported by the work of Liu and colleagues,[33] the radiomic signature seen on Dynamic Contrast Enhancement-MRI (DCE-MRI) can suggest the invasiveness of a tumor. Specifically, it was found that the DCE-MRI radiomic signature was an independent risk factor for lymphovascular invasion (odds ratio 2.895; $P = .031$). The presence of nodal disease and lymphovascular invasion identifies patients at higher risk for systemic disease and thus are candidates for neoadjuvant therapy. Based on preoperative evaluation, surgery may be rescheduled, with preference for early initiation of neoadjuvant therapy.

SUMMARY

Advances in breast cancer care over the past several decades have been marked by the development of a large array of therapeutic approaches, leading to multimodal therapy as part of an ever-expanding armamentarium of treatment options. However, much of what we offer in cancer therapy has significant treatment-associated sequelae. Furthermore, the treatment response by each tumor to any given treatment regimen can be highly variable. The good news is that recent developments in therapeutics are getting more and more targeted toward specific tumor-associated molecular defects. Such targeted therapies are generally more precise in their mechanism for tumor inhibition or destruction than traditional cytotoxic chemotherapy. In addition, our understanding of cancer biology continues to evolve. Through the use of multigene assays, molecular and expression profiling, and intrinsic subtyping, each tumor's growth as well as its likelihood to respond to a specific therapy is getting more precise. Together with "big data," such as biometrics gathered through the Internet of things, radiomics, and the rapid advances in high-throughput analysis, there is hope that the future of cancer therapy will continue to evolve toward a more precise approach. Through this improved precision can come greater predictability and efficacy of treatment individualized for each patient, while minimizing the risk of untoward side effects.

REFERENCES

1. Meisel JL, Venur VA, Gnant M, et al. Evolution of targeted therapy in breast cancer: where. Am Soc Clin Oncol Educ Book 2018;38:78–86.

2. Robert NJ. Clinical efficacy of tamoxifen. Oncology (Williston Park) 1997;11(2 Suppl 1):15–20.

3. Early Breast Cancer Trialists' Collaborative Group. Tamoxifen for early breast cancer: an overview of the randomised trials. Lancet 1998;351(9114):1451–67.

4. Schneider RE, Barakat A, Pippen J, et al. Aromatase inhibitors in the treatment of breast cancer in post-menopausal female patients: an update. Breast Cancer (Dove Med Press) 2011;3:113–25.

5. Mouridsen H, Gershanovich M, Sun Y, et al. Phase III study of letrozole versus tamoxifen as first-line therapy of advanced breast cancer in postmenopausal women: analysis of survival and update of efficacy from the international letrozole breast cancer group. J Clin Oncol 2003;21(11):2101–9.

6. Moja L, Compagnoni A, Brambilla C, et al. Trastuzumab containing regimens for metastatic breast cancer. In: Moja L, editor. Cochrane database of systematic reviews. Chichester (United Kingdom): John Wiley & Sons, Ltd; 2006. https://doi.org/10.1002/14651858.CD006242.

7. Nixon N, Verma S. A value-based approach to treatment of HER2-positive breast cancer: examining the evidence. Am Soc Clin Oncol Educ Book 2016;36:e56–63.

8. von Minckwitz G, Procter M, de Azambuja E, et al. Adjuvant pertuzumab and trastuzumab in early HER2-positive breast cancer. N Engl J Med 2017;377(2):122–31.

9. von Minckwitz G, Huang C-S, Mano MS, et al. Trastuzumab emtansine for residual invasive HER2-positive breast cancer. N Engl J Med 2018;380(7):617–28.

10. Baselga J, Campone M, Piccart M, et al. Everolimus in postmenopausal hormone-receptor–positive advanced breast cancer. N Engl J Med 2012;366(6): 520–9.

11. Jerusalem G, De Boer RH, Hurvitz S, et al. Everolimus plus exemestane vs everolimus or capecitabine monotherapy for estrogen receptor-positive, HER2-negative advanced breast cancer: the BOLERO-6 randomized clinical trial. JAMA Oncol 2018;4(10):1367–74.

12. Royce M, Bachelot T, Villanueva C, et al. Everolimus plus endocrine therapy for postmenopausal women with estrogen receptor-positive, human epidermal growth factor receptor 2-negative advanced breast cancer: a clinical trial. JAMA Oncol 2018;4(7):977–84.

13. Finn RS, Crown JP, Lang I, et al. The cyclin-dependent kinase 4/6 inhibitor palbociclib in combination with letrozole versus letrozole alone as first-line treatment of oestrogen receptor-positive, HER2-negative, advanced breast cancer (PALOMA-1/TRIO-18): a randomised phase 2 study. Lancet Oncol 2015;16(1):25–35.

14. Sledge GW, Toi M, Neven P, et al. MONARCH 2: abemaciclib in combination with fulvestrant in women with HR+/HER2-advanced breast cancer who had progressed while receiving endocrine therapy. J Clin Oncol 2017;35(25):2875–84.

15. Faraoni I, Graziani G. Role of BRCA mutations in cancer treatment with Poly(ADP-ribose) polymerase (PARP) inhibitors. Cancers (Basel) 2018;10(12):487.

16. Robson M, Im S-A, Senkus E, et al. Olaparib for metastatic breast cancer in patients with a germline BRCA mutation. N Engl J Med 2017;377(6):523–33.

17. Litton JK, Rugo HS, Ettl J, et al. Talazoparib in Patients with Adavanced Breast Cancer and a Germline BRCA Mutation. N Eng J Med 2018;379(8):753–63.

18. National Research Council. Toward precision medicine: building a knowledge network for biomedical research and a new taxonomy of disease. Washington, DC: National Academic Press; 2011.

19. Harris EER. Precision medicine for breast cancer: the paths to truly individualized diagnosis and treatment. Int J Breast Cancer 2018;2018:1–8.

20. Sørlie T, Perou CM, Tibshirani R, et al. Gene expression profiling can distinguish tumor subclasses of breast carcinomas. In: Hofmann W-K, editor. Gene expression profiling by microarrays, vol. 98. Cambridge (United Kingdom): Cambridge University Press; 2006. p. 132–61. https://doi.org/10.1017/CBO9780511545849.008.

21. Dai XF, Li T, Bai Z, et al. Breast cancer intrinsic subtype classification, clinical use, and future trends. Am J Cancer Res 2015;5(10):2929–43.

22. Koboldt DC, Fulton RS, McLellan MD, et al. The cancer genome atlas network. Nature 2012;490(7418):61–70.

23. Rouzier R, Perou CM, Symmans WF, et al. Breast cancer molecular subtypes respond differently to preoperative chemotherapy. Clin Cancer Res 2005; 11(16):5678–85.

24. Caudle AS, Yu T-K, Tucker SL, et al. Local-regional control according to surrogate markers of breast cancer subtypes and response to neoadjuvant chemotherapy in breast cancer patients undergoing breast conserving therapy. Breast Cancer Res 2012;14(3):R83.

25. Available at: https://www.cancer.gov/about-cancer/treatment/clinical-trials/nci-supported/nci-match. Accessed May 17, 2019.

26. Crivelli P, Ledda RE, Parascandolo N, et al. A new challenge for radiologists: radiomics in breast cancer. Biomed Res Int 2018;2018:1–10.

27. Fan M, Li H, Wang S, et al. Radiomic analysis reveals DCE-MRI features for prediction of molecular subtypes of breast cancer. PLoS One 2017;12(2):1–15.

28. Ma W, Zhao Y, Ji Y, et al. Breast cancer molecular subtype prediction by mammographic radiomic features. Acad Radiol 2019;26(2):196–201.
29. Drukker K, Li H, Antropova N, et al. Most-enhancing tumor volume by MRI radiomics predicts recurrence-free survival "early on" in neoadjuvant treatment of breast cancer. Cancer Imaging 2018;18(1):1–9.
30. Scoot JG, Berglund A, Schell MJ, et al. A Genome-based Model for Adjusting Radiotherapy Dose (GARD): a retrospective, cohort-based study. Lancet Oncology 2017;18(2):202–11.
31. Nguyen PL, Taghian AG, Katz MS, et al. Breast cancer subtype approximated by ER, PR, and Her2 receptors is associated with local-regional and distant failure after breast-conserving therapy. Int J Radiat Oncol 2007;69(3):S26.
32. Mazouni C, Rimareix F, Mathieu MC, et al. Outcome in breast molecular subtypes according to nodal status and surgical procedures. Am J Surg 2013;205(6): 662–7.
33. Liu Z, Feng B, Li C, et al. Preoperative prediction of lymphovascular invasion in invasive breast cancer with dynamic contrast-enhanced-MRI-based radiomics. J Magn Reson Imaging 2019;1–11. https://doi.org/10.1002/jmri.26688.

Precision Medicine in Pediatric Oncology

Kieuhoa T. Vo, MD, MAS[a], D. Williams Parsons, MD, PhD[b], Nita L. Seibel, MD[c],*

KEYWORDS

- Genomic profiling • Next-generation sequencing • Pediatric cancer
- Precision medicine • Targeted therapy

KEY POINTS

- The ultimate goal of precision medicine in pediatric oncology is to develop more effective and less toxic therapies in children, adolescents, and young adults with cancer.
- Precision clinical trials designed to assess the impact of molecularly targeted therapies in pediatric oncology are ongoing in the United States and Europe.
- Our understanding of the cancer genomic landscape, advancement in genomic technologies, and drug development in enhanced targeted therapies, may lead to future opportunities for precision medicine in pediatric oncology.

INTRODUCTION

Dramatic improvements in clinical outcomes have been seen for children and adolescents with cancer over the past 5 decades.[1] The improvement in survival is attributed primarily to risk-stratification of therapies and treatment intensification with cytotoxic chemotherapy and multimodal approaches. However, accelerating the progress of pediatric oncology requires both therapeutic advances and attention to diminishing the late effects of standard cytotoxic therapies. The ultimate goal of precision medicine in pediatric oncology is to develop more effective and less toxic therapies in children, adolescents, and young adults with cancer. With the advancement in diagnostic and molecular profiling technologies, precision medicine trials using clinical molecular

Disclosure: D.W. Parsons is the co-inventor on current and pending patents related to cancer genes discovered through sequencing of several adult cancer types and participates in royalty sharing related to those patents. The other authors have nothing to disclose.
a Department of Pediatrics, University of California San Francisco School of Medicine, Benioff Children's Hospital, 550 16th Street, 4th Floor, Box 0434, San Francisco, CA 94158, USA; b Section of Hematology/Oncology, Department of Pediatrics, Baylor College of Medicine, Texas Children's Hospital, 1102 Bates Avenue, Suite 1030.15, Houston, TX 77030, USA; c Division of Cancer Treatment and Diagnosis, Clinical Investigations Branch, National Cancer Institute, 9609 Medical Center Drive, 5W340, MSC9737, Bethesda, MD 20892, USA
* Corresponding author. National Cancer Institute, 9609 Medical Center Drive, 5W340, MSC9737, Bethesda, MD 20892, USA.
E-mail address: Seibelnl@mail.nih.gov

testing are becoming more common for adult malignancies. Similarly, there is an interest in how these technologies can be applied to tumors in children and adolescents to expand our understanding of the biology of pediatric cancers and evaluate the clinical implications of genomic testing for these patients, with the ultimate goal of improving survival for pediatric malignancies. This article reviews the early studies in pediatric oncology showing the feasibility of this approach, describes future plans to evaluate the clinical implications in multicenter clinical trials, and identifies the challenges of applying genomics in the patient population.

Feasibility of Precision Medicine in Pediatric Oncology

Biomarker-driven directed therapies have been used in pediatric oncology; however, combining this treatment approach with individualized genomic analysis is in its nascent phase.[2–4] Over the last 5 years, several pediatric oncology studies have explored the feasibility and use of genomics-driven precision medicine and provided the foundation for pursuing this approach. These pilot studies have explored different features of precision medicine and used various study designs, including patient population, timing of specimen acquisition, and inclusion of routine germline analysis. Of note, none of the published studies included prospective treatment arms as part of the study, although several studies include clinical follow-up to assess therapy response and outcomes to genomics-based recommendations.

The Baylor College of Medicine Advancing Sequencing in Childhood Cancer Care study completed enrollment of a primary cohort of 287 newly diagnosed and previously untreated patients with solid, including central nervous system (CNS), tumors.[5] Whole-exome sequencing (WES) was performed both on tumor samples and peripheral blood. In the report of the first 150 patients (<18 years), in whom 121 tumors were sequenced, 33 patients (27%) were found to have somatic mutations of established or potential clinical use. An additional 24 patients (20%) were found to have mutations in consensus cancer genes that were not classified as targetable. Diagnostic germline findings related to patient phenotype (either cancer or other diseases or both) were discovered in 15 (10%) of 150 cases, including 13 (8.6%) with pathogenic or likely pathogenic mutations in known cancer susceptibility genes. Treatment decisions or recommendations were not part of this study.

The University of Michigan Pediatric Michigan Oncology Sequencing study is modeled after the sequencing experience in adults with cancer.[6] The preliminary results of a cohort of 102 pediatric and young adult participants (25 years and younger) with refractory or relapsed cancer and newly diagnosed patients with high-risk or rare cancer types have been published.[6] Patients with both hematopoietic malignancies and solid tumors were included. A total of 91 patients underwent genomic analyses with WES of tumor and germline DNA, as well as RNA sequencing (RNA-seq) of tumor. A multidisciplinary tumor board provided clinical recommendations. They identified 42 patients (46%) with potentially actionable findings that were not identified by standard diagnostic tests, which did not include sequencing. Nine of the patients had germline findings, 10 had somatic actionable gene fusions found through RNA-seq, and 2 had their diagnosis changed because of the analyses. A total of 23 patients had an individualized care decision made based on either tumor or germline sequencing results. Fourteen of the patients had a change in therapy, 9 underwent genetic counseling, and 1 required both. Of the 14 patients, 9 had a clinical response to the change in therapy lasting more than 6 months. The median turnaround time for return of the results was 54 days.

The individualized cancer therapy (iCAT) study is a multicenter study led by investigators at the Dana-Farber Cancer Institute/Boston Children's Hospital to assess the feasibility of identifying actionable alterations and making individualized cancer therapy recommendations in pediatric and young adult patients (30 years and younger) with relapsed, refractory, or high-risk extracranial solid tumors.[7] A multidisciplinary expert panel reviewed the profiling results, and iCAT treatment recommendations were made if an actionable alteration was present, and an appropriate drug was available. Of the 100 participants, 31 had tumor submitted only from diagnosis, whereas the rest had tumor submitted from recurrence or local control or multiple specimens from recurrence and diagnosis. Tumor profiling was successful in specimens from 89 patients. Overall, 31 (31%) patients received an iCAT treatment recommendation and 3 received matched therapy. There were 0no objective responses. Three patients had a change in their diagnosis based on the tumor profiling. Six patients had an actionable alteration, but an appropriate drug was not available through a clinical trial or as a Food and Drug Administration (FDA)-approved therapy with an age-appropriate dose and formulation, and so an iCAT recommendation could not be made. Finally, 43 (43%) participants had results with potential clinical significance but not resulting in iCAT treatment recommendations were identified, including mutations indicating the possible presence of a cancer predisposition syndrome (if also found in the germline).

The Precision in Pediatric Sequencing Program at Columbia University Medical Center instituted a prospective clinical next-generation sequencing (NGS) for high-risk pediatric cancer and hematologic disorders.[8] WES and RNA-seq were performed on tumor and normal tissue from 101 high-risk pediatric patients. Results were initially reviewed by a molecular pathologist and subsequently by a multidisciplinary molecular tumor board. Potentially actionable alterations were identified in 38% of patients, of which 16% subsequently received matched therapy. In an additional 38% of patients, the genomic data provided clinically relevant information of diagnostic, prognostic, or pharmacogenomic significance. RNA-seq was clinically impactful in 37 of 65 patients (57%), providing diagnostic and/or prognostic information for 17 patients (26%) and identified therapeutic targets in 15 patients (23%). Known or likely pathogenic germline alterations were discovered in 18 of 90 patients (20%), with 14% having germline alternations in cancer predisposition genes. American College of Medical Genetics secondary findings were identified in 6 patients.

The Individualized Therapy for Relapsed Malignancies in Childhood project is a nationwide German program for children and young adults with refractory, relapsed cancers, which aims to identify therapeutic targets on an individualized basis.[9] In the report of the pilot phase, 57 patients aged 1 to 40 years with hematopoietic and solid malignancies were enrolled. Seven patients for whom no standard therapy was available were enrolled at the time of primary diagnosis. Tumor specimens were analyzed by WES, low-coverage whole-genome, and RNA-seq, as well as methylation and expression microarray analyses. A customized 7-step scoring algorithm was used to prioritize molecular targets and reviewed by an interdisciplinary molecular tumor board before returning the results to the treating physician. Germline DNA was screened on each patient for damaging alterations in a predefined list of known cancer predisposition genes. Turnaround time was 28 days. Of 52 patients, 26 (50%) with NGS data on their tumors harbored a potentially actionable alteration with a prioritization score of intermediate or higher. Ten patients received targeted therapy based on these results, with responses seen in some of the previously treated patients, although systematic follow-up was not an objective of this study. Underlying cancer predisposition was detected in 2 patients (4%). Comparative primary tumor–relapsed tumor analysis revealed substantial tumor evolution in addition to detection in one case of an unsuspected secondary malignancy.

The Institut Curie reported their 1-year experience of genetic analysis and molecular biology tumor board discussions for targeted therapies in pediatric solid tumors.[10] Tumor tissue from 60 pediatric patients (aged up to 21.5 years) with poor prognosis or relapsed or refractory solid, including CNS, tumors were analyzed with panel-based NGS and array comparative genomic hybridization. The most recently available tumor tissue was analyzed but, where there was inadequate material, a new biopsy was not requested and the initial diagnostic biopsy specimen was used. Recommendations from the molecular biology tumor board were given to the treating physicians. The mean turnaround time from patient referral to the molecular biology tumor board and release of results was 42 ± 16 days. Of the 58 patients in whom molecular profiling was feasible, 23 (40%) had a potentially actionable finding with high-grade gliomas having the highest number of targetable alterations. Of the 23 patients, 6 received a matched targeted therapy, with 5 being enrolled in a clinical trial and 1 by compassionate use. Two patients had a partial response. Despite having a targetable lesion, 4 patients could not receive therapy owing to lack of available clinical trials with the agents. The remaining 13 patients did not receive targeted therapy because of pursuit of conventional chemotherapy or change in health status. The investigators concluded that this approach is feasible, but only a small proportion of patients were able to receive the targeted therapy.

A single-institutional feasibility study (MOSCATO-01) at Gustave Roussy in France prospectively characterized genomic alterations in recurrent or refractory solid tumors of pediatric patients for selection of targeted therapy. Seventy-five patients underwent tumor biopsy or surgical resection of primary or metastatic tumor site on study. Tumor samples were analyzed by comparative genomic hybridization array NGS for 75 target genes, WES, and RNA-seq. Biological significance of the alterations and recommendation of targeted therapies available were discussed in a multidisciplinary tumor board. All patients were pretreated, 37% had CNS tumors, and 63% had an extracranial solid tumor. Successful molecular analysis in 69 patients detected an actionable alteration in various oncogenic pathways in 61% of patients, and a change in diagnosis was seen in 3 patients. Fourteen patients received 17 targeted therapies. This study demonstrated the feasibility of research biopsies in advanced pediatric malignancies for NGS and matching potential actionable mutations with targeted therapies.

These initial pilot studies demonstrated the feasibility of clinical sequencing for patients with childhood cancers and set the stage for subsequent precision medicine trials that prospectively assess the impact of molecularly targeted therapies in pediatric oncology. Our evolving understanding of the landscape of the cancer genome of pediatric cancers also necessitates the inclusion of unique genomic technologies, such as RNA analysis for fusion detection, and analyses of germline mutations for cancer susceptibility risk determination in forthcoming studies.

National Cancer Institute-Children's Oncology Group Pediatric Molecular Analysis for Therapeutic Choice: New Era of Precision Medicine in Pediatric Oncology

In collaboration with, and supported by, the National Cancer Institute (NCI), the Children's Oncology Group (COG) is leveraging the information gained from earlier precision medicine studies a step further in their design of a histology agnostic trial in which eligibility to treatment arms is determined based on predefined lists of genomic aberration(s), or actionable mutation(s) of interest (aMOI). Pediatric MATCH (Molecular Analysis for Therapeutic Choice) is a national clinical trial under a single IND (NCT03155620; Fig. 1). Relapsed tumor tissue from pediatric and young adult patients with recurrent or refractory tumors including CNS tumors, as well as lymphomas and histiocytic disorders, is submitted for molecular profiling. To provide broader access

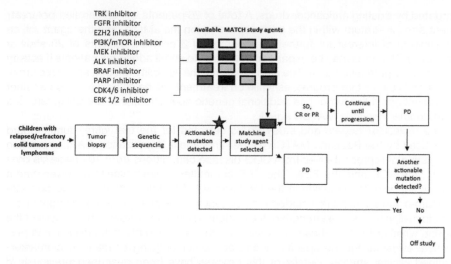

Fig. 1. NCI-COG Pediatric Molecular Analysis for Therapeutic Choice (MATCH) trial schema. ALK, anaplastic lymphoma kinase; CR, complete response; ERK, extracellular signal-regulated kinase; EZH2, enhancer of zeste homolog 2; FGFR, fibroblast growth factor receptor; PARP, poly-ADP ribose polymerase; PD, progressive disease; PI3K/mTOR, phosphoinositide 3-kinase/mammalian target of rapamycin; PR, partial response; SD, stable disease; TRK, tyrosine receptor kinase. (*From* Allen CE, Laetsch TW, Mody R, et al. Target and Agent Prioritization for the Children's Oncology Group-National Cancer Institute Pediatric MATCH Trial. *J Natl Cancer Inst.* 2017;109(5); with permission.)

to precision medicine trials for the adolescent and young adult oncology population, patients aged up to of 21 years are eligible to enroll on Pediatric MATCH.

Similar to the NCI MATCH study for adults, if an aberration is identified that has been defined as a driver mutation for a Pediatric MATCH study drug targeting the identified aberration, then the patient will have the opportunity to enroll onto the relevant single-agent treatment arm. Consequently, the trial is providing access to the study agent(s) for each patient in addition to tumor genomic analysis and treatment assignment. This trial will screen over 1000 patients for multiple targets and evaluate investigational targeted therapies for clinical activity in patients carrying specific mutations that can inform future trials. This is the largest pediatric oncology trial for all solid tumors to identify the molecular aberration(s) in the tumor and provide the investigational agent for the treatment of the identified molecular aberrations within the same trial. Similar to the NCI MATCH study for adults, Pediatric MATCH uses an analytically validated NGS-targeted assay of more than 4000 different mutations (single nucleotide variants, indels, copy-number alterations, and gene fusions) across more than 140 genes.[11] This type of basket or umbrella hybrid trial uses a rules-based treatment assignment, based on available preclinical and clinical data, which has not been used in the other pediatric trials.[12] This offers the advantage of predefining treatment based on the presence of a molecular aberration, ensures availability of agents within the context of a trial, and negates assignment bias because all patients with a predefined aMOI are assigned a given treatment.

The primary aims of the study are to determine the objective response rate in pediatric patients with advanced solid tumors and lymphomas harboring a priori specified genomic alterations treated with pathway-targeting agents, and to determine the proportion of pediatric patients whose tumors have pathway alterations that can be targeted by existing anticancer drugs. A total of 20 patients will be enrolled per treatment arm (or stratum within the arm) depending on the aMOIs, and the agent will be considered of interest for further development if 3 or more patients of 20 show a response. The arms may be expanded in the trial to enroll additional patients if activity is seen for a particular agent. The study will have the flexibility to open and close arms. A patient's tumor that progresses while on treatment will be eligible to go on another treatment arm if the tumor has additional genetic aberrations that are being targeted with another Pediatric MATCH agent.

The molecular targets and study drugs selected for the trial were identified and prioritized by the Pediatric MATCH Target and Agent Prioritization (TAP) committee consisting of representatives from COG disease committees from 10 children's hospitals, the NCI, and the FDA. The TAP committee systematically reviewed target and agent pairs for inclusion in the Pediatric MATCH trial. Criteria used to prioritize the target and agent pairs included the frequency of the alterations in the target in pediatric malignancies, the strength of the evidence linking the target to the activity of the agent, whether the target can be detected with the testing platform, clinical and preclinical evidence for the specific agent, and other ongoing or planned biomarker-defined clinical studies. Details of this process have been described previously.[13] Two criteria established for identifying specific agents to be considered for inclusion in Pediatric MATCH were demonstrated activity against tumors with a particular genomic alteration, and the establishment of an adult-recommended phase 2 dose. The same levels of evidence for drug selection used in NCI MATCH were applied for Pediatric MATCH.[11] Neither a completed pediatric phase 1 study nor a pediatric formulation was required to be considered for Pediatric MATCH trial. However, in the case of an oral agent, appropriately sized capsules or tablets were required to dose pediatric patients. Currently, the Pediatric MATCH trial has opened 10 treatment arms with the goal of investigating a total of 15 to 20 single agents based on ongoing review of new data and as agents become available based on the identified targets.

In a report of the first 422 patients enrolled from 93 COG sites on the Pediatric MATCH screening protocol, the median age is 13 years (range 1–21).[14] A tumor sample was submitted for 390 patients, sequencing was attempted for 370 patients (95%), and results were confirmed for 357 patients (92%). The median turnaround time for the tumor genomic results was 15 days. An aMOI for at least one of the 10 current treatment arms was identified in approximately 25% of patients with tumor submitted for the Pediatric MATCH screening protocol. These patients are assigned to a treatment arm and must meet the eligibility criteria to enroll on therapy.

There are some notable differences for Pediatric MATCH compared with NCI MATCH or similar precision medicine protocols. The number of molecular aberrations seen in pediatric tumors ($\sim$10%) is predicted to be much less than identified in adult malignancies.[15,16] These projections are based primarily on actionable mutation frequencies in newly diagnosed tumors. However, the Pediatric MATCH aMOI detection rate is currently higher than predicted.[14] In comparison, this Pediatric MATCH aMOI detection rate is higher than the match rate of for NCI MATCH for the first 10 treatment arms (approximately 9%).[11] One reason for this may be that patients with known targetable mutations from previous molecular testing are enrolling on the screening study at a higher rate on Pediatric MATCH. In addition, the Pediatric MATCH study is optimizing the chances of finding a targetable aberration in a patient's tumor by requiring the submission of tumor specimen from a biopsy done after recurrence or progression and as close to the time of genomic analysis, because tumors are likely to acquire more mutations over time.[17–20] In fact, in some studies in adults, it is recommended that a metastatic (as opposed to primary) lesion is biopsied.[21,22] To provide access for as many children and adolescents as possible, and because the risks associated with biopsies in children differ from adults, there is more flexibility with the timing of the biopsy (need not be obtained just before study enrollment as long as it is from a recurrence) or in the case of brain stem gliomas from the time of diagnosis in the Pediatric MATCH study. Finally, although tumors occurring in adults may have a larger number of mutations (on average), many of those mutations are passenger mutations that have been acquired over time and that may have little relevance to the biology (or treatment) of the tumor. Thus, the number of targetable mutations might be more similar in children and adults than initially projected based on total number of mutations.

Pediatric cancers harbor a different spectrum and frequency of mutations compared with adult cancers. For example, frequent targetable kinase alterations seen in lung cancer and breast cancer, such as EGFR and HER2, respectively, rarely occur in pediatric tumors. Therefore, such agents would not meet the selection criteria as treatment arms in Pediatric MATCH. Drug availability is another challenge, because agents are not yet available to target many of the recurrent aberrations identified in pediatric tumors. Based on the small number of pediatric cancers, and even smaller subgroups of molecular aberrations identified in the tumors, agents have not been developed to target some of the detectable molecular aberrations, such as epigenetic alterations.

Similar to several of the pediatric studies described earlier, germline DNA is collected and analyzed from all patients enrolled on Pediatric MATCH. In contrast, NCI MATCH does not evaluate germline molecular aberrations. By including germline analysis using the same panel as for tumor sequencing, it is possible to determine which mutations are of interest and which actionable mutations of interest represent germline variants in cancer susceptibility genes. Clinical genomics laboratories interpret the germline findings and provide a report back to the treating oncologist identifying whether any of the genomic aberrations included in the tumor sequencing report represent pathogenic or likely pathogenic germline variants in cancer susceptibility genes. The results of the germline analysis are not used for treatment assignment and are not meant to provide a comprehensive cancer susceptibility evaluation. However, based on the results, the treating pediatric oncologist may recommend formal genetic testing and counseling for the patient/family.

Other Precision Medicine Trials in Pediatric Oncology

There is a similar precision medicine initiative for the conduct of a genomically driven basket study for children and adolescents with relapsed or refractory cancers in Europe. The European Proof-of-Concept Therapeutic Stratification Trial of Molecular Anomalies in Relapsed or Refractory Tumors in Children uses genomic data derived from multiple panels from several ongoing sequencing studies in Europe.[23] In contrast to Pediatric MATCH, which uses predefined levels of evidence linking variants to targeted therapies, sequencing data are reviewed at a multidisciplinary molecular tumor board to determine whether an actionable variant is present and whether the variant is a match for one of the ESMART treatment arms or other targeted agent trials. At present, ESMART has 7 treatment arms for 5 genomic targets/pathways. Each of the treatment arms are conducted as individual clinical trials, with a phase 1 dose escalation phase and a phase 2 expansion phase. In contrast to Pediatric MATCH, which thus far includes only single agents, many of the treatment arms in ESMART combines targeted agents with chemotherapy.

The initial results for the European pediatric precision medicine initiative have been reported.[24] From 2016 to 2017, 174 patients with a median age of 13 years (range, 1–32) were included in the European molecular profiling trial (MAPPYACTS). Currently, the analysis for 104 patients has been completed. Seventy-six percent of patients had at least one "actionable" variant. Based on the detected alteration, 21 patients were included in the ESMART trial since it opened in August 2016, with 2 patients enrolling on 2 different treatment arms: CDK4/6 inhibitor ribociclib plus chemotherapy (1) or everolimus (5); DNA repair interfering combinations WEE1 inhibitor AZD1775 plus chemotherapy (4) and PARP inhibitor olaparib plus chemotherapy (1); dual mammalian target of rapamycin inhibitor vistusertib alone (1) or with chemotherapy (5); or nivolumab and cyclophosphamide (6).[24]

Umbrella trials focusing on specific diseases or histologies in pediatric oncology are currently underway in patients with relapsed and refractory or newly diagnosed cancers. These studies require a good understanding of the gene variants to be encountered in a specific diagnosis and its activity to targeted agents. Moreover, the feasibility of conducting these studies requires that the frequency of variants is sufficient to justify a clinical trial within a disease group. Examples of these studies are shown in **Table 1**.

A major challenge with these precision medicine clinical trials is that the treatment regimens are tailored to an increasingly smaller subset of genomically defined patients. Clinical trials such as these are intended to be screening trials to detect a signal in a histology agnostic cohort based on the genetic marker. Additional studies will

Table 1
Examples of the range of precision medicine trials in pediatric oncology

Study Design	Clinical Trial	Sponsor	NCT
Relapsed or refractory cancers			
Basket studies across multiple histologies	Pediatric MATCH	NCI-COG	
	AcSé-ESMART	Gustave Roussey	NCT02813135
Histology-specific umbrella studies	NEPENTHE (neuroblastoma)	CHOP	NCT02780128
	Ruxolitinib or Dasatinib + chemotherapy in Ph-like ALL	MD Anderson	NCT02420717
	RELPALL (ALL)	St. Jude	NCT03515200
Newly diagnosed cancers			
Histology-specific umbrella studies	Dasatinib + chemotherapy for Ph-like ALL	COG	NCT02883049
	Ruxolitinib + chemotherapy for CRLF2/JAK/STAT mutations in ALL	COG	NCT02723994
	Crizotinib + chemotherapy in ALK aberrant neuroblastoma	COG	NCT03126916
	Total therapy XVII JAK/STAT mutations in ALL/ lymphoma	St. Jude	NCT03117751
	Clinical/Molecular Risk-Directed Therapy in Medulloblastoma	St. Jude	NCT01878617
	BIOMEDE (DIPG)	Gustave Roussy	NCT02233049

Abbreviations: AcSé-ESMART, European Proof-of-Concept Therapeutic Stratification Trial of Molecular Anomalies in Relapsed or Refractory Tumors; ALK, anaplastic lymphoma kinase; ALL, acute lymphoblastic leukemia; CHOP, Children's Hospital of Philadelphia; COG, Children's Oncology Group; DIPG, diffuse intrinsic pontine glioma; NCT, ClinicalTrials.gov Identifier/Number.

need to be designed to assess the true activity of an agent in a prespecified cohort. Likewise, future study designs and statistical methods will need to address these issues as we analyze clinical trial results and consider incorporating this information into standard of care therapies.

SUMMARY

Molecular characterization has the potential to advance the management of pediatric cancer malignancies. The clinical integration of genome sequencing into standard clinical practice has been limited. Although there are still many obstacles remaining as precision medicine is applied to pediatric oncology, these studies represent the first step in exploring this application of genomic-directed treatment of patients with childhood cancer.

ACKNOWLEDGEMENT

Pediatric MATCH (APEC1621) is supported by NCTN Operations Center Grant U10CA180886 to the Children's Oncology Group from the National Cancer Institute of the National Institutes of Health.

REFERENCES

1. Siegel RL, Miller KD, Jemal A. Cancer statistics, 2016. CA Cancer J Clin 2016; 66(1):7–30.
2. Schultz KR, Bowman WP, Aledo A, et al. Improved early event-free survival with imatinib in Philadelphia chromosome-positive acute lymphoblastic leukemia: a children's oncology group study. J Clin Oncol 2009;27(31):5175–81.
3. Mosse YP, Lim MS, Voss SD, et al. Safety and activity of crizotinib for paediatric patients with refractory solid tumours or anaplastic large-cell lymphoma: a Children's Oncology Group phase 1 consortium study. Lancet Oncol 2013;14(6): 472–80.
4. Schultz KR, Carroll A, Heerema NA, et al. Long-term follow-up of imatinib in pediatric Philadelphia chromosome-positive acute lymphoblastic leukemia: Children's Oncology Group study AALL0031. Leukemia 2014;28(7):1467–71.
5. Parsons DW, Roy A, Yang Y, et al. Diagnostic yield of clinical tumor and germline whole-exome sequencing for children with solid tumors. JAMA Oncol 2016;2(5): 616–24.
6. Mody RJ, Wu YM, Lonigro RJ, et al. Integrative clinical sequencing in the management of refractory or relapsed cancer in youth. JAMA 2015;314(9):913–25.
7. Harris MH, DuBois SG, Glade Bender JL, et al. Multicenter feasibility study of tumor molecular profiling to inform therapeutic decisions in advanced pediatric solid tumors: the individualized cancer therapy (iCat) study. JAMA Oncol 2016; 2(5):608–15.
8. Oberg JA, Glade Bender JL, Sulis ML, et al. Implementation of next generation sequencing into pediatric hematology-oncology practice: moving beyond actionable alterations. Genome Med 2016;8(1):133.
9. Worst BC, van Tilburg CM, Balasubramanian GP, et al. Next-generation personalised medicine for high-risk paediatric cancer patients - The INFORM pilot study. Eur J Cancer 2016;65:91–101.
10. Pincez T, Clement N, Lapouble E, et al. Feasibility and clinical integration of molecular profiling for target identification in pediatric solid tumors. Pediatr Blood Cancer 2017;64(6). https://doi.org/10.1002/pbc.26365.

11. Conley BA, Gray R, Chen A, et al. Abstract CT101: NCI-molecular analysis for therapy choice (NCI-MATCH) clinical trial: interim analysis. Cancer Res 2016; 76(14 Supplement):CT101.

12. Takebe N, Yap TA. Precision medicine in oncology. Curr Probl Cancer 2017;41(3): 163–5.

13. Allen CE, Laetsch TW, Mody R, et al. Target and agent prioritization for the Children's Oncology Group-National Cancer Institute Pediatric MATCH trial. J Natl Cancer Inst 2017;109(5). https://doi.org/10.1093/jnci/djw274.

14. Parsons DW, Janeway KA, Patton D, et al. Identification of targetable molecular alterations in the NCI-COG Pediatric MATCH trial. J Clin Oncol 2019;37(suppl) [abstract: 10011].

15. Lawrence MS, Stojanov P, Polak P, et al. Mutational heterogeneity in cancer and the search for new cancer-associated genes. Nature 2013;499(7457):214–8.

16. Vogelstein B, Papadopoulos N, Velculescu VE, et al. Cancer genome landscapes. Science 2013;339(6127):1546–58.

17. Schleiermacher G, Javanmardi N, Bernard V, et al. Emergence of new ALK mutations at relapse of neuroblastoma. J Clin Oncol 2014;32(25):2727–34.

18. Eleveld TF, Oldridge DA, Bernard V, et al. Relapsed neuroblastomas show frequent RAS-MAPK pathway mutations. Nat Genet 2015;47(8):864–71.

19. Schramm A, Koster J, Assenov Y, et al. Mutational dynamics between primary and relapse neuroblastomas. Nat Genet 2015;47(8):872–7.

20. Padovan-Merhar OM, Raman P, Ostrovnaya I, et al. Enrichment of targetable mutations in the relapsed neuroblastoma genome. PLoS Genet 2016;12(12): e1006501.

21. Gerlinger M, Rowan AJ, Horswell S, et al. Intratumor heterogeneity and branched evolution revealed by multiregion sequencing. N Engl J Med 2012;366(10): 883–92.

22. Le Tourneau C, Kamal M, Tsimberidou AM, et al. Treatment algorithms based on tumor molecular profiling: the essence of precision medicine trials. J Natl Cancer Inst 2016;108(4). https://doi.org/10.1093/jnci/djv362.

23. Moreno L, Pearson ADJ, Paoletti X, et al. Early phase clinical trials of anticancer agents in children and adolescents - an ITCC perspective. Nat Rev Clin Oncol 2017;14(8):497–507.

24. Geoerger B, Schleiermacher G, Pierron G, et al. Abstract CT004: European pediatric precision medicine program in recurrent tumors: first results from MAPPYACTS molecular profiling trial towards AcSe-ESMART proof-of-concept study. Cancer Res 2017;77(13 Supplement):CT004.

Genomics Testing and Personalized Medicine in the Preoperative Setting

Rodney A. Gabriel, MD, MAS[a,b,]*, Brittany N. Burton, MHS[c],
Richard D. Urman, MD, MBA[d], Ruth S. Waterman, MD, MSc[e]

KEYWORDS

- Pharmacogenomics • Preoperative • Genetics • Outcomes • Opioids

KEY POINTS

- The application of pharmacogenomics principles in perioperative medicine is fairly novel and only a limited number of studies have shown its potential benefit in this clinical setting.

- Many enzymes are involved with the metabolism of various analgesic medications, leading to genetic variability, and consequently play a role in drug toxicity and efficacy. It seems logical that having pharmacogenomics information on patients before surgery would be a valuable tool to anesthesiologists because it would allow tailored and effective analgesic use in each patient.

- Challenges in executing pharmacogenomics programs into health care systems include physician buy-in and integration into usual clinical workflow, including the electronic health record.

- The preoperative testing clinic, a facility usually run by anesthesiologists and designed to screen patients for appropriateness of surgery, is an ideal location to perform pharmacogenomics screening.

This article was repurposed from Anesthesiology Clinics 36.4 (Preoperative Patient Evaluation-Zdravka Zafirova and Richard D. Urman).
Disclosure: R.A. Gabriel, R.S. Waterman, and R.D. Urman use CQuentia (Fort Worth, TX) for pharmacogenomics screening at their respective institutions.
[a] Division of Regional Anesthesia and Acute Pain, Department of Anesthesiology, University of California, San Diego, 200 W Arbor Dr, San Diego, CA 92103, USA; [b] Department of Medicine, Division of Biomedical Informatics, University of California, San Diego, 9500 Gilman Dr, La Jolla, CA 92093, USA; [c] School of Medicine, University of California, San Diego, 9500 Gilman Dr, La Jolla, CA 92093, USA; [d] Department of Anesthesiology, Perioperative and Pain Medicine, Harvard Medical School, Brigham and Women's Hospital, 75 Francis St, Boston, MA 02115, USA; [e] Department of Anesthesiology, University of California, San Diego, 200 W Arbor Dr, San Diego, CA 92103, USA
* Corresponding author. Department of Anesthesiology, University of California, San Diego, 9500 Gilman Drive, MC 0881, La Jolla, CA 92093-0881.
E-mail address: ragabriel@ucsd.edu

INTRODUCTION

Pharmacogenomics (PGx) is the study of how individuals' personal genotypes may affect their responses (phenotype) to various pharmacologic agents. The application of PGx principles in perioperative medicine is fairly novel and only a limited number of studies have shown its potential benefit in this clinical setting.[1-3] During a patient's perioperative experience, anesthesiology providers are tasked with the management of multimodal pharmacotherapy; these involve medications that are used to manage pain, prevent nausea and vomiting, induce and maintain anesthesia, provide muscle relaxation, and manage hemodynamics. Although the mechanisms of action of the many medications anesthesiologists use are to some degree understood, the precise effect a given dose will have on an individual may not be known until it is given. These inherent variations in response to medications are partly caused by PGx, a profile that is unique to each individual. Thus, in theory, having this personalized information for every patient planned to undergo surgery may aid in fine-tuning precision medicine when it comes to optimizing perioperative care.

Enhanced recovery after surgery (ERAS) pathways and perioperative surgical home (PSH) models are being widely adopted in an effort to protocolize evidence-based medicine systematically.[4] The goal is therefore to improve outcomes. Integration of PGx into such pathways may provide a huge step in optimizing care even further by having available additional information on patient-specific response to medications. Enhanced recovery pathways involve integral steps at all stages in a patient's perioperative journey, including:

1. Preadmission (ie, surgery clinic and preoperative care clinic)
2. Preoperative (ie, day of surgery before operation)
3. Intraoperative
4. Immediate postoperative (ie, recovery, physical therapy, nutrition, pain management)
5. Long-term postoperative phase (**Fig. 1**)

There are a variety of pharmacologic agents that are used at each stage of this perioperative process. Integration of PGx early in this process (ie, preadmission) may help providers practice precision medicine at all subsequent stages.

This article discusses the current evidence highlighting the potential of PGx with various drug categories used in the perioperative process and the challenges of integrating PGx into a health care system and relevant workflows.

PHARMACOGENOMICS AND PERIOPERATIVE MEDICATIONS

It is important to discuss the current evidence of PGx as it applies to various drug classes relevant to surgical patients; these include opioids, nonopioids, antiemetics, anticoagulants, and β-blockers. Much of anesthesiologists' clinical practice involves the titration of various drugs individualized to each patient.[2,3] Many enzymes are involved with the metabolism of various analgesic medications, leading to genetic variability, and consequently playing a role in drug toxicity and efficacy. It seems logical that having PGx information on patients before surgery would be a valuable tool to anesthesiologists because it would allow tailored and effective analgesic use in each patient. More studies are still needed to assess the effects of personalized dosing of anesthetics and analgesics during the perioperative process for various major surgeries.

Opioids

An individual's metabolism of opioids is largely determined by variations of cytochrome P (CYP) enzymes, including CYP2D6[5] and CYP3A4.[6,7] Studies have shown

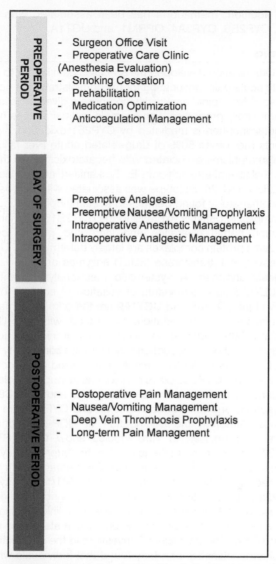

PREOPERATIVE PERIOD

- Surgeon Office Visit
- Preoperative Care Clinic (Anesthesia Evaluation)
- Smoking Cessation
- Prehabilitation
- Medication Optimization
- Anticoagulation Management

DAY OF SURGERY

- Preemptive Analgesia
- Preemptive Nausea/Vomiting Prophylaxis
- Intraoperative Anesthetic Management
- Intraoperative Analgesic Management

POSTOPERATIVE PERIOD

- Postoperative Pain Management
- Nausea/Vomiting Management
- Deep Vein Thrombosis Prophylaxis
- Long-term Pain Management

Fig. 1. Work flow of the perioperative process and how pharmacogenomics may be applied at each stage: preoperative, day of surgery, and postoperative phases.

variations in metabolism based on CYP2D6 for codeine,[8,9] tramadol,[10] and hydrocodone.[11] Morphine metabolism has been shown to be affected by canalicular multispecific organic anion transporter 2 (ABCC3),[12] organic cation transporter,[12] CYP2D6,[5] and P-glycoprotein transporter (encoded by ABCB1).[13] Adverse events related to morphine may also be affected by mu-receptor genotype (OPRM1).[14] Fentanyl metabolism can be affected by the CYP3A4 enzyme.[6,7] Furthermore, postoperative requirements for fentanyl have been associated with genotypes for catechol-O-methyltransferase (COMT) enzymes.[15] Tramadol metabolism may be affected by variations in CYP3A4, CYP2B6, CYP2D6, and various other transporter and receptor genes.[10] Hydromorphone metabolism is related to several types of

CYP genes.[16] In addition, methadone has been associated with several genes, including ABCB1, CYP2B6, CYP3A4, OPRM1, and UGT1A.[8,17–20]

Nonopioid Analgesics

The World Health Organization developed the so-called pain ladder to guide treatment of mild to moderate acute pain, advocating for the administration of nonopioid analgesics as the first step.[21] Nonopioid analgesics comprise a diverse class of medications that have antiinflammatory properties. For example, animal studies have shown that metabolism of acetaminophen is mediated by CYP2E1 oxidation.[22] Acetaminophen overdose represents more than 50% of drug-related acute liver failure, and studies have identified polymorphisms associated with hepatotoxicity.[23] In their investigation of 15 adults with thalassemia/hemoglobin E, Tankanitlert and colleagues[24] showed that the UGT1A6*2/UGT1A1*28 haplotype was associated with increased paracetamol concentrations. Another study found decreased acetaminophen glucuronide concentrations in urine samples in patients expressing the UGT2B15*2 variant.[25] Acetaminophen glucuronidation partial clearance and increased plasma concentration of acetaminophen plasma protein complexes are largely determined by UGT2B15*2 polymorphism.[26] Moreover, sulfotransferase (SULT) enzymes are involved in the sulfate conjugation of acetaminophen. A systematic meta-analysis identified SULT1A1, SULT1A2, and SULT1A3 as determinants of sulfation of acetaminophen.[27] Several studies have shown that UGT1A6 and UGT1A9 are the primary human allele variants mediating acetaminophen glucuronidation. Compared with the UGT1A6*1 allele variant, UGT1A6*2 had 60% higher acetaminophen glucuronidation activity.[28] However, for select human populations, a reduction in glucuronidation activity is observed with the UGTA1*28 isoform.[28] Ibuprofen is primarily metabolized by cytochrome enzymes and excreted into the urine. CYP2C9 plays a major role in ibuprofen clearance. Studies have shown that concomitant administration of ibuprofen and CYP2C9 inhibitors leads to drug-drug interactions and toxic effects. CY2C8 and CYP3A4 are also involved in ibuprofen clearance. Although the contribution of UDP-glucuronosyltransferases (UGTs) in vivo remains unclear, in vitro studies show that UGT1A3, UGT1A9, UGT2B7, and UGT2B17 glucuronidate ibuprofen to ibuprofen-acyl glucuronide.[29] Most studies have suggested a decrease in ibuprofen clearance with CYP2C9*3 polymorphism compared with individuals with the CYP2C9*1/*1 genotype.[29] Naproxen metabolism is mediated by UGT2B7 and CYP2C9 and interindividual genetic variations that lead to decreased metabolism of naproxen have been linked to higher risk of acute gastrointestinal hemorrhage.[30–32] Celecoxib is primarily metabolized by CYP2C9 and CYP3A4.[33,34] Prieto-Pérez and colleagues[33] investigated the association of CYP polymorphisms and pharmacokinetics and they found that individuals with CYP2C9*1/*3 and CYP2C9*3/*3 had lower celecoxib clearance compared with individuals with CYP2C9*1/*1. Chan and colleagues[35] evaluated cytochrome polymorphisms on colorectal adenoma recurrence in 1660 adult patients with colorectal cancer receiving celecoxib and found that patients who expressed CYP2C9*3 genotypes and received high-dose celecoxib had a lower risk of recurrence; however, this association was not found for patients with CYP2C9*2.

Benzodiazepines

It is well established that benzodiazepines primarily act on the central nervous system and are clinically used as sedative-anxiolytics and antiepileptics. In nerve cells, benzodiazepines facilitate ionotropic γ-aminobutyric acid (GABA) action by increasing the frequency of chloride channel opening. Metabolism of benzodiazepines is determined largely by oxidative metabolizing cytochrome enzymes, such as CYP3A4 and

CYP3A5, which are expressed primarily in the liver and intestine.[36] One study showed that CYP3A activity reflected clearance of urinary ratios of endogenous steroids, which was positively correlated with midazolam clearance.[36] Several studies have shown interindividual variability in CYP3A expression and activity, which influences the adverse effect profile.[37] It has been shown that midazolam is largely metabolized by CY3A4 and CYP3B to its active metabolite, 1'-hydroxymidazolam.[38] Miao and colleagues[37] found that CYP3A5*3, the most prevalent variant, was expressed in 85% to 95% of white people, 27% to 50% of African Americans, and 60% to 73% in Asian people. Further studies have shown that CYP3A4 290 A>G and CYP3Ab 22893 A>G allelic variants lead to reduced drug clearance.[39] In European and African American adults, CYP3A*5 was associated with 50% increase in enzyme induction.[39] The average population clearance of midazolam was shown to be 22% lower in patients with cancer expressing CYP3A5*3.[40] Increased midazolam concentrations and decreased metabolite ratios were observed in patients with cancer expressing CYP3A4*22, which is associated with decreased CYP3A4 activity.[41] Studies have shown that UGT1A4, UGT2B4, and UGT2B7 isoforms are primarily involved in glucuronide conjugation of midazolam metabolites.[42] After midazolam undergoes oxidative phosphorylation to its metabolite (ie, hydroxymidazolam) by CYP3A4, glucuronidated metabolites are produced by UDP-glucuronosyltransferases (UGTs) and ultimately excreted into the urine.[42] Studies have shown that variation in the response to lorazepam is determined largely by UGT2B15. In in vitro studies, ketoconazole was associated with inhibition of UGT2B7 glucuronidation of lorazepam.[43] The UGT1A1*28 variant has been shown to be associated with reduced elimination and consequently increased toxicity of lorazepam.[44]

Antiemetics

Ondansetron is a 5-hydroxytryptamine (5-HT3) serotonin antagonist and is used to prevent postoperative and chemotherapy-induced nausea and vomiting. Ondansetron has been shown to be metabolized by CYP3A4, CYP2D6, and CYP1A2.[45] The most common CYP2D6 variants of ondansetron metabolism may be divided into groups such as normal function (ie, CYP2D6*1 and *2), decreased function (ie, CYP2D6*9, *10, and *41), and no function (eg, CYP2D6*3–*6).[46] Individuals who express CYP2D6*2 are ultrametabolizers who experience treatment failure and therefore have increased risk of nausea and vomiting.[47] ATP-binding cassette (ABC) proteins are important in transport of ondansetron across cellular membranes. He and colleagues[48] evaluated 215 patients with acute myeloid leukemia with clinical resistance to ondansetron and found that the ABC subfamily B member 1 (ABCB1) transporter C3435T polymorphisms were associated with grade 3/4 vomiting. Moreover, ondansetron metabolism has been shown to be associated with hepatic organic cation transporter 1 (OCT1).[49] Although metoclopramide is partially metabolized by cytochromes, CYP2D6 is the primary determinant of metoclopramide metabolism. Parkman and colleagues[50] investigated the metoclopramide adverse effect profile in 100 adult patients with gastroparesis and found that patients with polymorphisms in CYP2D6 (ie, rs1080985, rs16947, rs3892097) and potassium voltage-gated channel subfamily H member 2 (KCNH2; ie, rs3815459) were more likely to experience side effects, however KCNH2 (ie, rs1805123) and ADRA1D (ie, rs2236554) polymorphisms were associated with a favorable clinical response. Although the exact antiemetic mechanism of action of dexamethasone is unclear, studies show that dexamethasone is involved in reduction in prostaglandin synthesis in the nervous system.[51] Expression of CYP2D6*3/*4/*5/*6 results in poor metabolism of haloperidol. As such, these individuals are at risk of increased risk for QT prolongation and arrhythmias.[47] In their evaluation of novel loci associated with the response to antipsychotic medication, Yu and colleagues[52] found several polymorphisms associated with an increased risk of psychotic disorders and response to antipsychotic medications. CYP2D6 has been shown to be associated with metabolism of promethazine.[53] Moreover, CYP2D6 polymorphisms have been shown to be associated with H1 antihistamine–induced sedation.[54]

Anticoagulants

Anticoagulation is prescribed for a wide range of conditions, including, but not limited to, atrial fibrillation, acute coronary syndrome, pulmonary embolism, deep venous thrombosis, and cerebrovascular accident. It is well established that warfarin, which is most widely used in the prevention of venous thromboembolism and cerebrovascular accident in patients with atrial fibrillation, is metabolized by CYP2C9 and vitamin K epoxide reductase complex (VKORC1).[55] Studies have shown that CYP 2C9*2, CYP 2C9*3, and VKORC1 A haplotype warfarin polymorphisms are associated with slower metabolism.[55] The antiplatelet activity of clopidogrel has been shown to reduce the risk of vascular disease.[56] Roughly 25% of individuals treated with clopidogrel experience treatment failure, and studies have shown that CYP2C9 and CYP2C19 are involved in the metabolism of clopidogrel.[56] Polymorphism in ATP-Binding Cassette Subfamily B Member 1 (ABCB1), Paraoxonase-1 (PON1), Carboxyl Esterase 1 (CES1), and P2Y12 receptors are associated with clopidogrel metabolism.[56]

β-Blockers

Metoprolol is a β_1-adrenoreceptor antagonist and is often prescribed to manage myocardial infarction, supraventricular tachycardia, hypertension, and heart failure. Blocking adrenergic receptors reduces heart rate and contractility. Although there are more than 100 identified polymorphisms of CYP2D6, studies have shown that CYP2D6 is responsible for 70% to 80% of metoprolol metabolism. The wide genetic variation in CYP2D6 for metoprolol and carvedilol has been shown to lead to variation in clinical response. Individuals may be classified as poor, intermediate, extensive, and ultrarapid metoprolol or carvedilol metabolizers.[57,58] Studies have shown that CYP2D6 nonexpressors have roughly a 5-fold increase in plasma concentrations of metoprolol and consequently decreased cardioselectivity and increased risk of adverse effects.[59,60] As such, ultrarapid metabolizers are at risk of treatment failure, whereas poor metabolizers may experience toxic adverse effects. Gao and colleagues[59] evaluated 319 patients who received metoprolol succinate for heart rate control following percutaneous coronary intervention and found that CYP2D6*10 polymorphisms were associated with a lower heart rate. As such, metoprolol guidelines have been published to recommend dosing adjustments and requirements based on CYP2D6 polymorphisms.[47] Carvedilol is also commonly prescribed to treat hypertension and heart failure.[58] Luzum and colleagues[57] assessed the relationship of CYP2D6 polymorphisms and maintenance does of metoprolol and carvedilol. Patients with CY2D6*4 had lower and higher maintenance dose requirements for metoprolol and carvedilol, respectively.

Local Anesthetics

Common local anesthetics used in the perioperative period include lidocaine, bupivacaine, ropivacaine, and mepivacaine. Their primary site of action is neuronal sodium channels. Few studies have shown any clinical correlation between genomics and response to local anesthetics. Lidocaine and bupivacaine are metabolized by CYP3A4, whereas ropivacaine is metabolized by CYP1A2.[38] Furthermore, patients with MC1R variants have decreased response to lidocaine.[61]

Malignant Hyperthermia

Malignant hyperthermia (MH) is a rare and potentially life-threatening autosomal dominant inherited condition associated with inhaled anesthetics or succinylcholine. Roughly 50% of MH cases are associated with ryanodine receptors (RYRs) or calcium voltage-gated channels (CACNA1S).[62] RYR and CACNA1S polymorphisms have been identified in families with multiple cases of MH.[63] Genetics variations in RYR1 account for roughly 80% of all cases of MH, whereas polymorphisms of CACNA1S have been shown to account for less than 1% of MH cases.[64] Preoperative PGx information for RYRs would be useful in determining which patients should not receive succinylcholine or volatile anesthetics.

INTEGRATION INTO PERIOPERATIVE WORKFLOW

Although PGx is not new, its widespread implementation into perioperative care is still at its infancy. Challenges in executing such programs include physician buy-in and integration into usual clinical workflow, including the electronic health record (EHR).[1] To facilitate physician buy-in would require more published data reporting both the prevalence of genetic risk to various perioperative medications and definitive outcomes associated with tailoring medications based on PGx. Integration into clinical work flow is also key and would require a collaboration between health care providers and the informatics department to create useful and user-friendly interfaces and alerts that may lead to improved execution of PGx. In order to obtain more universal adoption of perioperative PGx, there needs to be:

1. More high-quality evidence that surgical outcomes improve with PGx
2. Easy-to-access and user-friendly interfaces integrated into electronic medical record systems
3. Protocols put into place that allow PGx to easily fit into regular clinical workflow

More High-Quality Evidence that Surgical Outcomes Improve with Pharmacogenomics

Integration of PGx-guided therapy for surgical patients has potential to improve outcomes; however, more large-scale definitive studies are required. To date, there have been some small-scale cohort studies reporting its impact.[2,3] In one cross-sectional study, approximately 150 patients with postoperative trauma were analyzed and genetic associations of OPRM1 and COMT and postoperative pain/opioid consumption were made. The investigators concluded that OPRM1 and COMT may contribute to the variability of opioid consumption.[65] Other studies have shown that there is no genetic association of various genes with fentanyl consumption in gynecologic patients[66] and obstetric patients.[67] Several studies, as described earlier, have shown associations between different genes and postoperative opioid use.[65–77] However, studies are now needed that focus on PGx interventions and postoperative outcomes. Senagore and colleagues[68] conducted a study whose methodology involved comparing results with historical controls in patients undergoing colorectal resections or ventral hernia repair and showed improvement in opioid consumption. The investigators produced a guided analgesic protocol based on the assessment of 6 CYP, COMT, OPRM1, and ABCB1 genes. Depending on the patients' genotypes, analgesics were dose adjusted or avoided as appropriate. Large-scale prospective randomized controlled trials are needed to prove its efficacy.

Easy-to-Access and Easy-to-Understand Interfaces Integrated into Electronic Medical Record Systems

Because there are several genes that have already been implicated in perioperative medication metabolism, a complete list of genetic interactions with pharmacologic agents may prove to be too long and complex for the average health care provider to review. Therefore, the interface presenting this information should be strategically designed. Specifically, integrating known PGx polymorphisms into ERAS protocols could prove to be the most useful for the health care provider.

Protocols Put into Place that Allow Pharmacogenomics to Easily Fit into Regular Clinical Workflow

The perioperative work flow needs to be an efficient process while maintaining patient safety. PGx screening results should be transferred directly into EHR systems and should contain some of these components: (1) customized report generation depending on provider and institution preferences; (2) data tracking and analytics; (3) easy-to-use provider-facing interface in the record explaining the key salient results for each patient as well as a separate section with more detailed information; and (4) EHR-integrated real-time alerts associated with genetic risks. On a daily operating room schedule integrated into the EHR, patients who have PGx screening available are identified by a unique icon next to their names. The presence of this icon alerts providers that results are available in the EHR. **Fig. 2**A is an example screenshot of 1 component of a patient's test results, listing each gene screened and the metabolism status of that gene. Based on the genes tested, providers are given information regarding potential drug responses to different pharmacologic categories, including anticoagulation, beta-blockade, sedatives, antiemetics, hypnotics, muscle relaxants, analgesics (opioid and nonopioids), and volatile anesthetics. **Fig. 2**B and C are example screenshots of a patient's thrombosis profile summary and response to analgesic medications, respectively.

WHEN TO PERFORM PHARMACOGENOMICS SCREENING

The time at which to perform PGx screening must take into consideration the time required to obtain the final results in relation to when the patient's surgery is scheduled. In addition, there must be an appropriate amount of allocated time to consent and educate the patient regarding PGx. The preoperative testing clinic (a facility usually run by anesthesiologists and designed to screen patients for appropriateness of surgery) is an ideal location to perform such tasks. At that time, health care providers can perform preoperative behavioral and medical risk assessments to determine appropriateness of PGx testing. Patients at risk for opioid dependence or pharmacologically associated adverse events can be recognized early and PGx may be used to potentially optimize perioperative care. Furthermore, genetics do not change and results may be used for multiple subsequent surgical encounters.

SUMMARY

The use of PGx to personalize perioperative care is promising, but there are several challenges that must be met before this becomes a widespread practice. This article discusses studies in the basic and clinical science showing the association of various genes and response to perioperative medications, both opioid and nonopioid medications. However, more evidence needs to be generated by high-quality large-scale randomized controlled trials to show efficacy and cost-effectiveness. Furthermore, protocols need to be developed that guide perioperative providers on how to

A

Genetic Summary

Gene	Result	Activity
CYP2C19	*1/*17	Rapid metabolizer
CYP2C9	*1/*3	Intermediate metabolizer
CYP2D6	*1/*2	Extensive metabolizer
CYP3A4	*1/*1	Extensive metabolizer
CYP3A5	*3/*3	Poor metabolizer
DPYD	*1/*1	Extensive metabolizer
TPMT	*1/*1	Extensive metabolizer
Factor V Leiden (F5)	Normal	See Thrombosis Profile (Pg. 4)
Prothrombin (F2)	Normal	See Thrombosis Profile (Pg. 4)
MTHFR (A1298C)	Heterozygous	See Thrombosis Profile (Pg. 4)
MTHFR (C677T)	Heterozygous	See Thrombosis Profile (Pg. 4)

B

Thrombosis Profile

Tested Genes (Alleles)	Genotype	Predicted Phenotype	Clinical Guidance
Prothrombin (F2)	Normal	Normal risk expected based on the patient's genotype.	The absence of these variant alleles of Prothrombin (Factor 2) and Factor V Leiden suggests that the patient does not have the elevated risk of thrombosis associated with these genetic markers.
Factor V Leiden	Normal		
MTHFR (A1298C)	Heterozygous		
MTHFR (C677T)	Heterozygous		

C

Drug	Finding	Recommendation	Evidence
NSAIDs			
Celecoxib	*Intermediate metabolizer* CYP2C9 *1/*3	Patients with this CYP2C9 metabolism status who are treated with celecoxib may have an increased risk of gastrointestinal bleeding as compared to patients with the wild-type (*1/*1) genotype.	
	AGT rs699 A/A (WT)	Patients with this genotype may have increased likelihood of acute coronary syndrome when exposed to NSAIDs compared to patients with the homozygous genotype.	
Diclofenac	*Intermediate metabolizer* CYP2C9 *1/*3	Patients with this CYP2C9 metabolism status who are treated with diclofenac may have an increased risk of gastrointestinal bleeding as compared to patients with the wild-type (*1/*1) genotype.	
	AGT rs699 A/A (WT)	Patients with this genotype may have increased likelihood of acute coronary syndrome when exposed to NSAIDs compared to patients with the homozygous genotype.	
Opioids			
Codeine	*Extensive metabolizer* CYP2D6 *1/*2	The genotype predicts that the patient is an Extensive Metabolizer for Codeine. Consider label recommended dosage of Codeine if no contraindication.	
Hydrocodone	*Extensive metabolizer* CYP2D6 *1/*2	The genotype predicts that the patient is an Extensive Metabolizer for Hydrocodone. Consider label recommended dosage of Hydrocodone if no contraindication.	
Methadone	CYP2B6 rs3745274 G/T (HET)	Consider label recommended dosage of Methadone if no contraindication.	
Oxycodone	*Extensive metabolizer* CYP2D6 *1/*2	Consider label recommended dosage of Oxycodone if no contraindication.	

Fig. 2. Example screenshots of a pharmacogenomics tool integrated into the EHR. (*A*) A patients' metabolism status to various genes. (*B*) A patient's thrombosis profile based on pharmacogenomics. (*C*) A patient's response to various analgesics based on pharmacogenomics. (*Courtesy of* CQuentia, Fort Worth, TX.)

interpret genetic testing findings in terms of medication dose adjustment. There is a plethora of results that may be generated from a single PGx screening (especially if there are hundreds/thousands of genes tested), but a detailed presentation of these results to a provider may prove to be useless given the fast-paced nature of the operating room. The presentation of results must be strategically designed so that it proves functional to the providers. In addition, clinical decision support could be integrated into such systems to help improve PGx implementation into the perioperative space. The centerpiece to meet these challenges involves EHR integration, because this is the key to minimally disturbing the clinical flow, easing the visualization and execution of the results to physicians (eg, automated alerts/notifications, clinical decision support, and data visualization), while contributing to the cost-effectiveness of PGx testing.

REFERENCES

1. Gabriel RA, Ehrenfeld JM, Urman RD. Preoperative genetic testing and personalized medicine: changing the care paradigm. J Med Syst 2017;41(12):185.
2. Saba R, Kaye AD, Urman RD. Pharmacogenomics in pain management. Anesthesiol Clin 2017;35(2):295–304.
3. Saba R, Kaye AD, Urman RD. Pharmacogenomics in anesthesia. Anesthesiol Clin 2017;35(2):285–94.
4. Beverly A, Kaye AD, Ljungqvist O, et al. Essential elements of multimodal analgesia in enhanced recovery after surgery (ERAS) guidelines. Anesthesiol Clin 2017;35(2):e115–43.
5. Linares OA, Fudin J, Schiesser WE, et al. CYP2D6 phenotype-specific codeine population pharmacokinetics. J Pain Palliat Care Pharmacother 2015;29(1):4–15.
6. Tateishi T, Krivoruk Y, Ueng YF, et al. Identification of human liver cytochrome P-450 3A4 as the enzyme responsible for fentanyl and sufentanil N-dealkylation. Anesth Analg 1996;82(1):167–72.
7. Feierman DE, Lasker JM. Metabolism of fentanyl, a synthetic opioid analgesic, by human liver microsomes. Role of CYP3A4. Drug Metab Dispos 1996;24(9):932–9.
8. Armstrong SC, Cozza KL. Pharmacokinetic drug interactions of morphine, codeine, and their derivatives: theory and clinical reality, part I. Psychosomatics 2003;44(2):167–71.
9. Crews KR, Gaedigk A, Dunnenberger HM, et al. Clinical pharmacogenetics implementation consortium (CPIC) guidelines for codeine therapy in the context of cytochrome P450 2D6 (CYP2D6) genotype. Clin Pharmacol Ther 2012;91(2):321–6.
10. Lassen D, Damkier P, Brosen K. The pharmacogenetics of tramadol. Clin Pharmacokinet 2015;54(8):825–36.
11. Hutchinson MR, Menelaou A, Foster DJ, et al. CYP2D6 and CYP3A4 involvement in the primary oxidative metabolism of hydrocodone by human liver microsomes. Br J Clin Pharmacol 2004;57(3):287–97.
12. Venkatasubramanian R, Fukuda T, Niu J, et al. ABCC3 and OCT1 genotypes influence pharmacokinetics of morphine in children. Pharmacogenomics 2014; 15(10):1297–309.
13. Sadhasivam S, Chidambaran V, Zhang X, et al. Opioid-induced respiratory depression: ABCB1 transporter pharmacogenetics. Pharmacogenomics J 2015; 15(2):119–26.
14. Chidambaran V, Mavi J, Esslinger H, et al. Association of OPRM1 A118G variant with risk of morphine-induced respiratory depression following spine fusion in adolescents. Pharmacogenomics J 2015;15(3):255–62.

15. Zhang F, Tong J, Hu J, et al. COMT gene haplotypes are closely associated with postoperative fentanyl dose in patients. Anesth Analg 2015;120(4):933–40.

16. Benetton SA, Borges VM, Chang TK, et al. Role of individual human cytochrome P450 enzymes in the in vitro metabolism of hydromorphone. Xenobiotica 2004; 34(4):335–44.

17. Bunten H, Liang WJ, Pounder DJ, et al. OPRM1 and CYP2B6 gene variants as risk factors in methadone-related deaths. Clin Pharmacol Ther 2010;88(3):383–9.

18. Bunten H, Liang WJ, Pounder D, et al. CYP2B6 and OPRM1 gene variations predict methadone-related deaths. Addict Biol 2011;16(1):142–4.

19. Hodges LM, Markova SM, Chinn LW, et al. Very important pharmacogene summary: ABCB1 (MDR1, P-glycoprotein). Pharmacogenet Genomics 2011;21(3):152–61.

20. Kharasch ED, Hoffer C, Whittington D, et al. Role of hepatic and intestinal cytochrome P450 3A and 2B6 in the metabolism, disposition, and miotic effects of methadone. Clin Pharmacol Ther 2004;76(3):250–69.

21. Carlson CL. Effectiveness of the World Health Organization cancer pain relief guidelines: an integrative review. J Pain Res 2016;9:515–34.

22. Lee SS, Buters JT, Pineau T, et al. Role of CYP2E1 in the hepatotoxicity of acetaminophen. J Biol Chem 1996;271(20):12063–7.

23. Yoon E, Babar A, Choudhary M, et al. Acetaminophen-induced hepatotoxicity: a comprehensive update. J Clin Transl Hepatol 2016;4(2):131–42.

24. Tankanitlert J, Morales NP, Howard TA, et al. Effects of combined UDP-glucuronosyltransferase (UGT) 1A1*28 and 1A6*2 on paracetamol pharmacokinetics in beta-thalassemia/HbE. Pharmacology 2007;79(2):97–103.

25. Navarro SL, Chen Y, Li L, et al. UGT1A6 and UGT2B15 polymorphisms and acetaminophen conjugation in response to a randomized, controlled diet of select fruits and vegetables. Drug Metab Dispos 2011;39(9):1650–7.

26. Court MH, Zhu Z, Masse G, et al. Race, gender, and genetic polymorphism contribute to variability in acetaminophen pharmacokinetics, metabolism, and protein-adduct concentrations in healthy African-American and European-American volunteers. J Pharmacol Exp Ther 2017;362(3):431–40.

27. Yamamoto A, Liu MY, Kurogi K, et al. Sulphation of acetaminophen by the human cytosolic sulfotransferases: a systematic analysis. J Biochem 2015;158(6):497–504.

28. Mazaleuskaya LL, Sangkuhl K, Thorn CF, et al. PharmGKB summary: pathways of acetaminophen metabolism at the therapeutic versus toxic doses. Pharmacogenet Genomics 2015;25(8):416–26.

29. Mazaleuskaya LL, Theken KN, Gong L, et al. PharmGKB summary: ibuprofen pathways. Pharmacogenet Genomics 2015;25(2):96–106.

30. Sullivan-Klose TH, Ghanayem BI, Bell DA, et al. The role of the CYP2C9-Leu359 allelic variant in the tolbutamide polymorphism. Pharmacogenetics 1996;6(4):341–9.

31. Bowalgaha K, Elliot DJ, Mackenzie PI, et al. S-Naproxen and desmethylnaproxen glucuronidation by human liver microsomes and recombinant human UDP-glucuronosyltransferases (UGT): role of UGT2B7 in the elimination of naproxen. Br J Clin Pharmacol 2005;60(4):423–33.

32. Agundez JA, Garcia-Martin E, Martinez C. Genetically based impairment in CYP2C8- and CYP2C9-dependent NSAID metabolism as a risk factor for gastrointestinal bleeding: is a combination of pharmacogenomics and metabolomics required to improve personalized medicine? Expert Opin Drug Metab Toxicol 2009;5(6):607–20.

33. Prieto-Pérez R, Ochoa D, Cabaleiro T, et al. Evaluation of the relationship between polymorphisms in CYP2C8 and CYP2C9 and the pharmacokinetics of celecoxib. J Clin Pharmacol 2013;53(12):1261–7.

34. Wang B, Wang J, Huang SQ, et al. Genetic polymorphism of the human cyto-chrome P450 2C9 gene and its clinical significance. Curr Drug Metab 2009; 10(7):781–834.

35. Chan AT, Zauber AG, Hsu M, et al. Cytochrome P450 2C9 variants influence response to celecoxib for prevention of colorectal adenoma. Gastroenterology 2009;136(7):2127–36.e1.

36. Shin KH, Choi MH, Lim KS, et al. Evaluation of endogenous metabolic markers of hepatic CYP3A activity using metabolic profiling and midazolam clearance. Clin Pharmacol Ther 2013;94(5):601–9.

37. Miao J, Jin Y, Marunde RL, et al. Association of genotypes of the CYP3A cluster with midazolam disposition in vivo. Pharmacogenomics J 2009;9(5):319–26.

38. Cohen M, Sadhasivam S, Vinks AA. Pharmacogenetics in perioperative medi-cine. Curr Opin Anaesthesiol 2012;25(4):419–27.

39. Floyd MD, Gervasini G, Masica AL, et al. Genotype-phenotype associations for common CYP3A4 and CYP3A5 variants in the basal and induced metabolism of midazolam in European- and African-American men and women. Pharmacoge-netics 2003;13(10):595–606.

40. Seng KY, Hee KH, Soon GH, et al. CYP3A5*3 and bilirubin predict midazolam population pharmacokinetics in Asian cancer patients. J Clin Pharmacol 2014; 54(2):215–24.

41. Elens L, Nieuweboer A, Clarke SJ, et al. CYP3A4 intron 6 C>T SNP (CYP3A4*22) encodes lower CYP3A4 activity in cancer patients, as measured with probes mid-azolam and erythromycin. Pharmacogenomics 2013;14(2):137–49.

42. Seo KA, Bae SK, Choi YK, et al. Metabolism of 1'- and 4-hydroxymidazolam by glucuronide conjugation is largely mediated by UDP-glucuronosyltransferases 1A4, 2B4, and 2B7. Drug Metab Dispos 2010;38(11):2007–13.

43. Sawamura R, Sato H, Kawakami J, et al. Inhibitory effect of azole antifungal agents on the glucuronidation of lorazepam using rabbit liver microsomes in vitro. Biol Pharm Bull 2000;23(5):669–71.

44. Herman RJ, Chaudhary A, Szakacs CB. Disposition of lorazepam in Gilbert's syn-drome: effects of fasting, feeding, and enterohepatic circulation. J Clin Pharma-col 1994;34(10):978–84.

45. Dixon CM, Colthup PV, Serabjit-Singh CJ, et al. Multiple forms of cytochrome P450 are involved in the metabolism of ondansetron in humans. Drug Metab Dispos 1995;23(11):1225–30.

46. Bell GC, Caudle KE, Whirl-Carrillo M, et al. Clinical Pharmacogenetics Implemen-tation Consortium (CPIC) guideline for CYP2D6 genotype and use of ondansetron and tropisetron. Clin Pharmacol Ther 2017;102(2):213–8.

47. MacKenzie M, Hall R. Pharmacogenomics and pharmacogenetics for the inten-sive care unit: a narrative review. Can J Anaesth 2017;64(1):45–64.

48. He H, Yin JY, Xu YJ, et al. Association of ABCB1 polymorphisms with the efficacy of ondansetron in chemotherapy-induced nausea and vomiting. Clin Ther 2014; 36(8):1242–52.e2.

49. Tzvetkov MV, Saadatmand AR, Bokelmann K, et al. Effects of OCT1 polymor-phisms on the cellular uptake, plasma concentrations and efficacy of the 5-HT(3) antagonists tropisetron and ondansetron. Pharmacogenomics J 2012; 12(1):22–9.

50. Parkman HP, Mishra A, Jacobs M, et al. Clinical response and side effects of metoclopramide: associations with clinical, demographic, and pharmacogenetic parameters. J Clin Gastroenterol 2012;46(6):494–503.

51. Perwitasari DA, Gelderblom H, Atthobari J, et al. Anti-emetic drugs in oncology: pharmacology and individualization by pharmacogenetics. Int J Clin Pharm 2011; 33(1):33–43.

52. Yu H, Yan H, Wang L, et al. Five novel loci associated with antipsychotic treatment response in patients with schizophrenia: a genome-wide association study. Lancet Psychiatry 2018;5(4):327–38.

53. Nakamura K, Yokoi T, Inoue K, et al. CYP2D6 is the principal cytochrome P450 responsible for metabolism of the histamine H1 antagonist promethazine in human liver microsomes. Pharmacogenetics 1996;6(5):449–57.

54. Saruwatari J, Matsunaga M, Ikeda K, et al. Impact of CYP2D6*10 on H1-antihistamine-induced hypersomnia. Eur J Clin Pharmacol 2006;62(12): 995–1001.

55. Li J, Wang S, Barone J, et al. Warfarin pharmacogenomics. P T 2009;34(8):422–7.

56. Brown SA, Pereira N. Pharmacogenomic impact of CYP2C19 variation on clopidogrel therapy in precision cardiovascular medicine. J Pers Med 2018; 8(1) [pii:E8].

57. Luzum JA, Sweet KM, Binkley PF, et al. CYP2D6 genetic variation and beta-blocker maintenance dose in patients with heart failure. Pharm Res 2017;34(8): 1615–25.

58. Lymperopoulos A, McCrink KA, Brill A. Impact of CYP2D6 genetic variation on the response of the cardiovascular patient to carvedilol and metoprolol. Curr Drug Metab 2015;17(1):30–6.

59. Gao X, Wang H, Chen H. Impact of CYP2D6 and ADRB1 polymorphisms on heart rate of post-PCI patients treated with metoprolol. Pharmacogenomics 2017. https://doi.org/10.2217/pgs-2017-0203.

60. Dean L. Metoprolol therapy and CYP2D6 genotype. In: Pratt V, McLeod H, Dean L, et al, editors. Medical genetics summaries. Bethesda (MD): National Center for Biotechnology Information (US); 2012.

61. Liem EB, Joiner TV, Tsueda K, et al. Increased sensitivity to thermal pain and reduced subcutaneous lidocaine efficacy in redheads. Anesthesiology 2005; 102(3):509–14.

62. Kim JH, Jarvik GP, Browning BL, et al. Exome sequencing reveals novel rare variants in the ryanodine receptor and calcium channel genes in malignant hyperthermia families. Anesthesiology 2013;119(5):1054–65.

63. Muniz VP, Silva HC, Tsanaclis AM, et al. Screening for mutations in the RYR1 gene in families with malignant hyperthermia. J Mol Neurosci 2003;21(1):35–42.

64. Gonsalves SG, Ng D, Johnston JJ, et al. Using exome data to identify malignant hyperthermia susceptibility mutations. Anesthesiology 2013;119(5):1043–53.

65. Khalil H, Sereika SM, Dai F, et al. OPRM1 and COMT gene-gene interaction is associated with postoperative pain and opioid consumption after orthopedic trauma. Biol Res Nurs 2017;19(2):170–9.

66. Kim KM, Kim HS, Lim SH, et al. Effects of genetic polymorphisms of OPRM1, ABCB1, CYP3A4/5 on postoperative fentanyl consumption in Korean gynecologic patients. Int J Clin Pharmacol Ther 2013;51(5):383–92.

67. Landau R, Liu SK, Blouin JL, et al. The effect of OPRM1 and COMT genotypes on the analgesic response to intravenous fentanyl labor analgesia. Anesth Analg 2013;116(2):386–91.

68. Senagore AJ, Champagne BJ, Dosokey E, et al. Pharmacogenetics-guided analgesics in major abdominal surgery: further benefits within an enhanced recovery protocol. Am J Surg 2017;213(3):467–72.

69. De Gregori M, Diatchenko L, Ingelmo PM, et al. Human genetic variability contributes to postoperative morphine consumption. J Pain 2016;17(5):628–36.
70. Ren ZY, Xu XQ, Bao YP, et al. The impact of genetic variation on sensitivity to opioid analgesics in patients with postoperative pain: a systematic review and meta-analysis. Pain Physician 2015;18(2):131–52.
71. Henker RA, Lewis A, Dai F, et al. The associations between OPRM 1 and COMT genotypes and postoperative pain, opioid use, and opioid-induced sedation. Biol Res Nurs 2013;15(3):309–17.
72. Boswell MV, Stauble ME, Loyd GE, et al. The role of hydromorphone and OPRM1 in postoperative pain relief with hydrocodone. Pain Physician 2013; 16(3):E227–35.
73. Ochroch EA, Vachani A, Gottschalk A, et al. Natural variation in the mu-opioid gene OPRM1 predicts increased pain on third day after thoracotomy. Clin J Pain 2012;28(9):747–54.
74. De Gregori M, Garbin G, De Gregori S, et al. Genetic variability at COMT but not at OPRM1 and UGT2B7 loci modulates morphine analgesic response in acute postoperative pain. Eur J Clin Pharmacol 2013;69(9):1651–8.
75. Bartosova O, Polanecky O, Perlik F, et al. OPRM1 and ABCB1 polymorphisms and their effect on postoperative pain relief with piritramide. Physiol Res 2015; 64(Suppl 4):S521–7.
76. Hayashida M, Nagashima M, Satoh Y, et al. Analgesic requirements after major abdominal surgery are associated with OPRM1 gene polymorphism genotype and haplotype. Pharmacogenomics 2008;9(11):1605–16.
77. Zwisler ST, Enggaard TP, Mikkelsen S, et al. Lack of association of OPRM1 and ABCB1 single-nucleotide polymorphisms to oxycodone response in postoperative pain. J Clin Pharmacol 2012;52(2):234–42.

Individualizing Care
Management Beyond Medical Therapy

Laura Cristoferi, MD[a], Alessandra Nardi, PhD[b], Pietro Invernizzi, MD, PhD[a],
George Mells, MRCP, PhD[c], Marco Carbone, MD, PhD[a,d,*]

KEYWORDS

- Primary biliary cholangitis • Precision medicine • Risk-stratification
- Autoimmune liver disease • Individualized care • Novel therapies • Omics

KEY POINTS

- The forthcoming availability of several novel drugs in primary biliary cholangitis (PBC) coupled with the rise of high-throughput omics technologies prompt changing the paradigm of the management of the disease.
- Precision medicine (PM), through the application of omics-based approaches, should enable identifying disease variants, stratifying patients according to disease trajectory, risk of disease progression, and likelihood of response to different therapeutic options in PBC.
- The development of PM needs specific interventions, such as sequencing more genomes, creating bigger biobanks, and linking biological information to health data in electronic medical record.
- The authors envisage that a diagnostic work-up of PBC patients will include information on genetic variants and molecular signature that may define a particular subtype of disease and provide an estimate of treatment response and survival.

Primary biliary cholangitis (PBC) is a chronic, autoimmune liver disease characterized by nonsuppurative granulomatous cholangitis, causing progressive duct destruction and portal fibrosis that progresses slowly to biliary cirrhosis. A substantial proportion of cases eventually develops cirrhosis with attendant complications, such as portal hypertension, chronic liver failure, or hepatocellular cancer (HCC). PBC, therefore, remains a leading indication for liver transplantation (LT).

This article was repurposed from Clinics in Liver disease 22.3 (Primary Biliary Cholangitis- Elizabeth J. Carey and Cynthia Levy).
The authors have nothing to disclose.
[a] Division of Gastroenterology and Hepatology, Department of Medicine and Surgery, University of Milan Bicocca, Piazza dell'Ateneo Nuovo, 1, 20126 Milan, Italy; [b] Department of Mathematics, Tor Vergata University of Rome, Via della Ricerca Scientifica 1, Rome, Italy; [c] Academic Department of Medical Genetics, University of Cambridge, Hills Road 1, Cambridge, UK; [d] Academic Department of Medical Genetics, University of Cambridge, Cambridge, UK
* Corresponding author. Division of Gastroenterology and Hepatology, Department of Medicine and Surgery, University of Milan Bicocca, Piazza dell'Ateneo Nuovo, 1, 20126 Milan, Italy.
E-mail address: marco.carbone@unimib.it

Advances over the past several years have improved the ability to individualize care in PBC. This is prescient: individualizing care is the aim of precision medicine (PM), described as "an emerging approach for disease treatment and prevention that takes into account individual variability in genes, environment, and lifestyle for each person."[1] The aim of PM is to enable health care workers and biomedical researchers to more accurately predict which treatment and prevention strategies for a particular disease will work in which groups of patients. It contrasts with a 1-size-fits-all approach, in which disease treatment and prevention strategies are developed for the average patient, with less consideration for interindividual variation.[1]

PM relies on biomarkers (or panels of biomarkers) that accurately predict key outcomes, such as treatment response or disease progression (**Fig. 1**). Biomarkers may be measurements in blood, urine, saliva, or other biofluids—but the concept also encompasses features on imaging and histology. Omics-based approaches, coupled with computational and bioinformatics methods, provide an unprecedented opportunity to accelerate biomarker discovery. Such approaches include genetic analysis (genome-wide genotyping of common to rare variants, exome sequencing, and whole-genome sequencing) and a plethora of approaches for profiling the epigenome, transcriptome, proteome, and metabolome (**Fig. 2**). PM is applicable to PBC, as it is to other chronic inflammatory conditions, especially now with the current and forthcoming availability of more efficacious medications.

The clinical features and investigations that already enable individualizing the care of PBC patients are reviewed—and how emerging biomedical technologies might improve the ability to individualize management of PBC patients in the future is speculated on. The premise throughout is that individualized care for PBC, current or future, should achieve the following major objectives:

- Identification of disease variants that may require different management, such as PBC with autoimmune features or the premature ductopenic variant

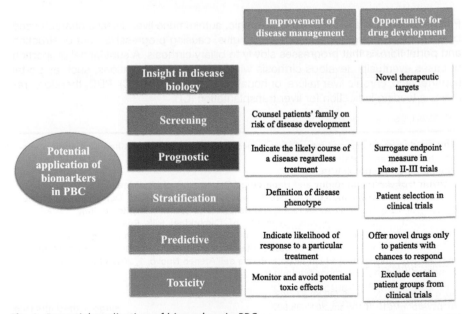

Fig. 1. Potential application of biomarkers in PBC.

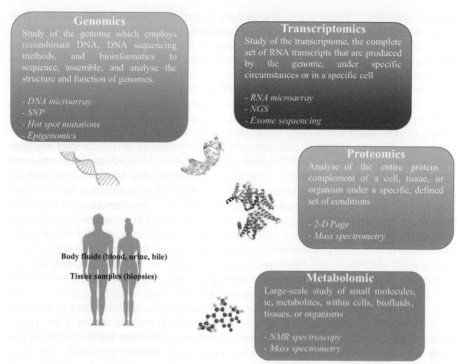

Fig. 2. Example of omics platforms available to study PBC. DNA, deoxyribonucleic acid; NGS, next-generation sequencing; NMR, nuclear magnetic resonance; RNA, ribonucleic acid.

- Stratification of patients according to different disease trajectories that might require different forms of surveillance, such as portal hypertensive progression; hepatocellular failure-type progression, or progression to HCC
- Stratification based on the risk of disease progression
- Stratification based on the likelihood of response to, and side-effects from, different therapeutic options.

In each case, stratification should ideally reflect the underlying mechanism because this informs ongoing development or repurposing of pharmacotherapies. Beyond these major objectives, the authors anticipate that PM initiatives will identify hitherto unknown disease subphenotypes.

STRATIFICATION OF DISEASE VARIANTS

Clinical variants with different disease course have been described. It remains unclear whether these clinical entities are distinct conditions (resulting from unique pathologic processes) or extremes of phenotype (resulting from shared pathologic processes). Either way, it is important to identify patients with variant syndromes because they have different disease trajectories and benefit from different management. PM initiatives should provide insight, if carefully designed.

Primary Biliary Cholangitis with Features of Autoimmune Hepatitis

Also known as PBC/autoimmune hepatitis (AIH) overlap syndrome, primary biliary cholangitis with features of autoimmune hepatitis is a variant of PBC in which there are characteristics of both PBC and AIH. Features of AIH coexist in 8% to 10% of patients with PBC.[2] There is ongoing debate about the nature of PBC with AIH features, whether it is simply the presence of 2 disorders (ie, PBC and AIH) in one individual, a distinct condition with characteristics of PBC and AIH, or one end of the spectrum of hepatic activity in PBC. One reason for ongoing debate is that interface hepatitis, a hallmark of AIH, is also common in PBC, albeit less florid and without other, characteristic histologic features of AIH, such as rosetting and emperipolesis.

It is important to recognize PBC with AIH features because patients with this variant are likely to benefit from combined treatment with ursodeoxycholic acid (UDCA) and classic immunosuppression. Without immunosuppression, it is associated with earlier development of liver fibrosis and cirrhosis.[3] A diagnosis of PBC with AIH features should be considered in any PBC patient with moderately to highly elevated transaminases, with or without raised IgG. The diagnosis should also be considered in PBC patients with inadequate response to treatment with UDCA treatment after 6 months to 12 months showing elevated transaminases[2] (other than elevated alkaline phosphatase [ALP]). The diagnosis is currently made according to Paris criteria[4] endorsed by the European Association for the Study of the Liver (EASL)[2] (**Box 1**). It follows that a liver biopsy is mandatory to make a diagnosis. For those who satisfy the Paris criteria, international guidelines on PBC[2] recommend treatment with immunosuppression (combined or sequential treatment with corticosteroids and azathioprine) in the short term and medium term. A potential problem with the Paris criteria, however, is that they were developed without tests of specificity or sensitivity. This is not a criticism: there is no gold standard against which the Paris criteria may be tested. They might, however, be specific at the cost of sensitivity, meaning they may fail to identify all patients who could benefit from immunosuppression in addition to UDCA. The most recent EASL guidelines on AIH[5] recommend immunosuppressive treatment of AIH patients at lower cutoffs for transaminase or IgG levels and a modified histologic activity index as low as 4 of 18 points. A trial of glucocorticosteroids may, therefore, be warranted in PBC patients with prominent interface hepatitis demonstrated on liver biopsy, even if they do not fulfill the Paris criteria for diagnosis of overlap.

The authors' practical approach is to focus the treatment on the disease that seems to be the predominant entity. The authors suggest treating with immunosuppression if

---

Box 1
Diagnostic criteria of primary biliary cholangitis–autoimmune hepatitis overlap syndrome

PBC criteria

ALP >2 × ULN or GGT >5 × ULN

AMA >1:40

Liver biopsy specimen showing florid bile duct lesions

AIH criteria

ALT >5 × ULN or a positive test for anti–smooth muscle antibodies

IgG >2 × ULN

Liver biopsy showing moderate or severe periportal or periseptal lymphocytic piecemeal necrosis

Diagnostic criteria of PBC-AIH overlap syndrome of which at least 2 of 3 accepted criteria for PBC and AIH, respectively, should be present. Histologic evidence of moderate to severe lymphocytic piecemeal necrosis (interface hepatitis) is mandatory for the diagnosis.

Data from Chazouillères O, Wendum D, Serfaty L, et al. Primary biliary cirrhosis-autoimmune hepatitis overlap syndrome: clinical features and response to therapy. Hepatology 1998;28(2):296–301.

histology shows moderate to severe interface hepatitis, regardless of biochemical (transaminases) activity. Also, the authors suggest not overdiagnosing overlap presentations, given the common presence of mildly to moderately raised transaminases associated with cholestasis (likely a surrogate marker of the interface hepatitis that the authors observe associated with the florid duct lesions of PBC) and that generally responds well to choleretic agents.

Better characterization of PBC with features of AIH is a priority for PM initiatives. The aim is to identify PBC patients who would benefit from immunosuppression, ideally at diagnosis and ideally without recourse to a liver biopsy. Transcriptomic analysis of liver tissue might identify transcriptional biomarkers that can then be sought in circulation. RNA sequencing is not well suited for diagnostic use due to its complexity, computational intensity, limited throughput, and need for expert technicians. In addition, it is challenging to perform RNA sequencing analyses with small amounts of tissue, especially formalin-fixed paraffin-embedded (FFPE) biopsies, which is a limiting factor in large-scale studies. Transcriptomic analysis can be performed on FFPE biopsies using the NanoString (South Lake Union, Seattle, WA, USA) nCounter platform analyzing total mRNA level of hundreds of genes. This might highlight the expression of regulatory genes encoding essential inflammatory chemokines, interleukin, complement that might offer a signature of treatment response to immunosuppressive therapy.[6] Tissue markers should then be correlated with circulating markers. An approach that might yield suitably accurate circulating biomarkers includes immunoassays based on Luminex (Austin, Texas) xMAP (multianalyte profiling) technology that enable simultaneous detection and quantitation of multiple secreted proteins (cytokines, chemokines, growth factors, and so forth).[7] This high-throughput technology produces results comparable to ELISA but with greater efficiency, speed, and dynamic range, allowing a correlation of the composition of the portal tract infiltrate and transcriptomics readout with peripheral immune-phenotype before and after immunosuppression therapy.

The relevant studies will not, however, be easy. PBC with AIH features is a rare variant of a rare disease; therefore, recruiting an adequately powered sample will be difficult. Potential biomarkers must be tested against the current standard, which, as discussed previously, might be flawed. The study would require liver biopsy of PBC patients without AIH features; this is unlikely to be popular among support groups. Potential biomarkers must be tested against biochemical and histologic response to immunosuppression.

Premature Ductopenic Variant

The premature ductopenic variant is a poorly described variant of PBC, with only 4 cases reported in the literature.[8] It is defined histologically by extreme ductopenia disproportionate to the extent of liver fibrosis. Although the extent of fibrosis may be limited initially, progression to cirrhosis might be inevitable in the long term. Laboratory tests show a marked elevation of cholestatic markers (ALP and gamma glutamyl transferase [GGT]). The bilirubin may be elevated without features cirrhosis or portal hypertension. Owing to markedly decreased quality of life, LT is generally required within a few years of presentation.

Whether this is a disease variant or an extreme form of PBC is unknown. When this variant is suspected, a liver biopsy is required to confirm the diagnosis. This may be useful to inform prognosis and guide management. Patients with this variant typically develop jaundice early in the disease course. As a result, they may satisfy listing criteria for LT before they have cirrhosis and liver failure. Provided the symptoms of cholestasis are adequately controlled, however, LT may be safely deferred. Conversely, pruritus is severe and notoriously difficult to control in this variant. For PBC patients known to have premature ductopenia, it may be appropriate to progress rapidly through the stepwise treatment of cholestatic pruritus and consider LT for quality of life sooner rather than later.

There is no specific therapy for the premature ductopenic variant. Anecdotally, response to UDCA is often poor. The efficacy of obeticholic acid and off-label medications, such as fibrates and budesonide, is untested. Clinicians may be hesitant to offer obeticholic acid, which may exacerbate pruritus, to a patient with severe itch. This has to be weighed, however, against the potential benefit of bile duct regeneration and future symptoms improvement. However this approach has not been proved yet.

PM might have a major role to define this severe variant and highlight pathways of treatment.

In the hypothesis that these patients have different bile acid (BA) pools that are increased in their hydrophobicity beyond the capacity of UDCA to moderate or atypical patterns of handling of UDCA itself, a first approach might be to study the phenotype and quantity of circulating BA and liver tissue BA using mass spectrometry–based targeted metabolomics approach. A major challenge, however, is to select patients with this rare condition for study; this implies a major collaborative national or international effort to identify patients with severe itch and jaundice who should then undergo liver biopsy for confirmation diagnosis.

STRATIFICATION OF PATIENTS BY DIFFERENT DISEASE TRAJECTORIES

Preliminary data suggest there may be different patterns of disease progression in PBC. The Japanese Society of Hepatology describes 3 clinical types (**Fig. 3**). A majority of patients progress gradually and remain in the asymptomatic stage for longer than a decade (gradual progressive type). Some patients who progress to portal hypertension presenting without jaundice (portal hypertension type) and others progress rapidly to

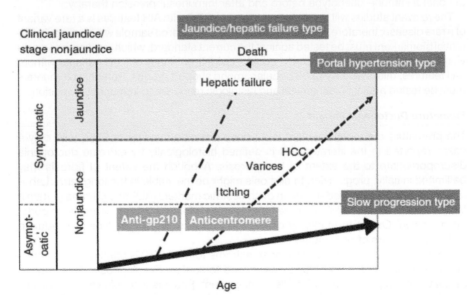

Fig. 3. Potential trajectories based on the autoantibody profile in PBC. (*From* Working Subgroup (English version) for Clinical Practice Guidelines for Primary Biliary Cirrhosis. Guidelines for the management of primary biliary cirrhosis: the Intractable Hepatobiliary Disease Study Group supported by the Ministry of Health, Labour and Welfare of Japan. Hepatol Res 2014;44 Suppl S1:71–90; with permission.)

jaundice and ultimately hepatic failure (jaundice/hepatic failure type). The jaundice/hepatic failure type tends to affect relatively younger patients compared with the other 2 types. Patients with the jaundice/hepatic failure–type PBC are often positive for anti-gp210 antibody, whereas those with the portal hypertension–type PBC have anticentromere antibodies. The latter antibodies are characteristic of systemic sclerosis (SSc) but are also found in PBC patients without coexistent SSc.[9–11] The only two, old, studies describing this clinical entity looking at the underlying pathologic damage suggest that portal hypertension is initially of presinusoidal type and then as the disease progresses is joined by a sinusoidal component.[12,13] Alternatively, given the strong association with anticentromere antibodies, the mechanism might be that of noncirrhotic portal hypertension occurring in SSc and other connective tissue diseases. As a form of noncirrhotic portal hypertension, this type of progression of PBC is generally recognized by (1) the presence of unequivocal signs of portal hypertension; (2) the absence of cirrhosis, advanced fibrosis, or other causes of chronic liver diseases; and (3) the absence of thrombosis of the hepatic veins or of the portal vein at imaging. In these patients, the liver function is usually preserved; the treatment is based on the monitoring and prevention of complications of portal hypertension, with only few patients requiring LT for unmanageable portal hypertension or liver failure. A target proteomic approach looking at markers on inflammation and/or fibrosis and their dynamic over time might be appropriate to better define different disease trajectories.

STRATIFICATION OF PATIENTS BY RISK OF DISEASE PROGRESSION
Stage of Disease

Measures of liver fibrosis, that is, the stage of disease, are relevant in prognostication because in PBC; as in other liver diseases, they predict treatment response and liver failure.[14,15] Liver biopsy is the gold standard to assess liver fibrosis. Its invasiveness with significant potential complications and the poor patient acceptance, however, coupled with its inherent shortcomings related to sampling error have led to an exponential interest in the identification and use of noninvasive markers of liver fibrosis. To be included in clinical practice, noninvasive markers should predict treatment response, survival, and the risk of cancer and portal hypertension.

Pathologic features

Liver biopsy for staging of PBC lost favor after the publication of a study by Garrido and Hubscher[16]: in this study, the investigators evaluated fibrosis using Menghini needle from simulated needle biopsy in fields approximately the size of conventional needle biopsy and from whole-section scanning in areas with little and extensive fibrosis. They showed considerable variation in the stage of fibrosis across each of 50 explanted PBC livers, evaluated using the staging system of Ludwig and colleagues.[17] There have been no subsequent studies to verify or challenge this observation. There is less variability in staging using the new system of Nakanuma.[18] In this system, the stage of disease is based on the degree of fibrosis, bile duct loss, and cholestasis assessed by deposition of orcein-positive granules, whereas the grade of necroinflammatory activity is based on cholangitis, interface hepatitis, and lobular hepatitis. The accumulation of orcein-positive granules occurs evenly across the PBC liver, which means that staging using the Nakanuma system is more reliable.[19,20] Even so, the widespread availability of noninvasive measures of fibrosis means that liver biopsy for staging of PBC is somewhat obsolete. Liver biopsy does, however, remain useful in certain settings. Nowadays, the main indications are to confirm the diagnosis of PBC when PBC-specific antibodies are absent and confirm a diagnosis of PBC with AIH features. Liver biopsy is also useful to confirm ductopenia and assess the relative contribution of each liver injury when a comorbid liver disease is present, such as nonalcoholic steatohepatitis. In patients with inadequate response to UDCA, liver biopsy may provide the explanation. For example, it may identify a previously unsuspected variant syndrome, steatohepatitis, or interface hepatitis of moderate or greater severity.

Liver biopsy could undoubtedly inform risk stratification in PBC. For example, the Nakanuma[18] stage and grade have been shown to correlate with clinicolaboratory features. Recent data have shown an association between interface hepatitis, bridging fibrosis, and cirrhosis and long-term outcomes in PBC independently from UDCA treatment, confirming historical data.[14,15] Furthermore, the presence of ductopenia/bile duct loss has been reported to be a predictor of PBC progression.[21] These data suggest that liver biopsy could be as important for treatment stratification in PBC as it is in AIH and other liver conditions—but the balance of risk versus benefit and patient acceptability need to be considered. This is exactly the area of unmet need that PM should address.

Ideally, analysis of circulating byproducts (eg, epigenetic factors, such as micro-RNAs, cell-free DNA, glucose, and fatty acid and amino acid metabolites from high-throughput omics profiling, among others), namely liquid biopsy, could provide access to molecular information related to the severity of portal inflammation, biliary damage, cholestasis, and fibrosis and thus improve patients' stratification and allow evaluation of disease biology dynamically over time. To develop such noninvasive surrogate test of liver pathology, a major effort would be required to select a cohort of PBC patients who undergo deep phenotyping of liver tissue samples and biofluids (such as serum, plasma, peripheral blood mononuclear cells, and urine) at different time points. Building up a well-sized cohort in such a rare condition and performing follow-up liver biopsies are challenging. Nonetheless, this is a promising horizon toward which further research efforts should be directed.

Non-invasive markers of fibrosis

Liver stiffness measure (LSM) by transient elastography, aspartate aminotransferase (AST)-to-platelet ratio index (APRI), and enhanced liver fibrosis (ELF) represent alternative and potentially complementary approaches to assessing liver fibrosis and are associated with minimal discomfort and hazard to the patient when compared with biopsy.

LSM has been regarded as a good marker to exclude or confirm severe fibrosis or cirrhosis in PBC. The largest study (N = 103) demonstrated high specificity and sensitivity (>90%) of transient elastography in distinguishing severe fibrosis from cirrhosis in PBC patients.[22] A threshold of LSM greater than 9.6 kPa (F4) at diagnosis was associated with a 5-fold increase in the risk of future liver decompensation or LT. The results were not as strong when it came to intermediate fibrosis (F2: sensitivity 0.67, specificity 1.0). This may be due to the presence of inflammation and cholestasis that could overestimate the measurement.[22]

Investigators also show a predictive role of longitudinal assessment of LSM: a progression of greater than or equal to 2.1 kPa/y in the overall cohort was associated with 8-fold increased risk of liver decompensation, LT, or death.[22] Before proposing regular assessments of LSM as standard practice, however, for example, on an annual basis, these data would require external validation in a large cohort, in longitudinal fashion. Also, whether the risk estimate is independent of the achievement of treatment response has to be clarified.

There is convincing evidence for the use of APRI in prognostication of PBC. In a recent study of 386 PBC patients, the APRI measured at baseline or after 1 year of therapy with UDCA independently predicted LT-free survival. Measured at baseline, APRI greater than 0.54 best discriminated good versus poor prognosis. Measured after 1 year of treatment, APRI greater than 0.54 identified a subgroup of patients at risk of disease progression despite meeting the Paris I, Paris II, Barcelona, and Toronto definitions of UDCA response.[23]

The ELF score, calculated from serum measurements of hyaluronic acid, tissue inhibitor of metalloproteinase 1, and procollagen type III N-terminal propeptide, is another noninvasive marker proposed in PBC. There is only 1 multicenter study (N = 161) looking at the ELF score in PBC. ELF showed a good ability to stratify patients into groups of differing prognoses. Prediction of decompensations was good, with an area under a receiver operating characteristic curve (AUC) ranging between 0.68 and 0.78 based on how many years before the first event the serum was collected; however, no calibration, that is, agreement between predicted versus observed events, was provided.[24]

The development of the ELF score is paradigmatic of the potentiality to transfer biomarkers (proteomic markers, in this case) from discovery to clinical practice; it also highlights the pitfalls and limitations of this. Despite encouraging results, ELF score has not been adopted with enthusiasm in clinical practice in PBC, and overall in hepatology, and its use is currently limited to clinical trials where fibrosis is an endpoint (eg, https://clinicaltrials.gov/ct2/show/NCT01672853). The main limitation for its use include the high cost of the equipment and the need for regular recalibration and trained operators to ensure accuracy and reproducibility of the results. There are also concerns regarding its biological meaning and interpretation: for instance, it is unclear whether ELF is a marker of disease severity or disease stage; fluctuations over time have not been studied and this prevents its application as dynamic biomarker; also, stratified analysis for influence factors, such as gender, age and ethnicity, are lacking.[25] More data on ELF score application in patients with PBC are needed to make firm recommendations on its use in this condition A head-to-head comparison with the most robust, currently available prognostic tests, such as the continuous scoring systems (UK-PBC and GLOBE scores) and the transient elastography, would be of interest.

Treatment Response Profile

First-line treatment of PBC is UDCA.[26] Although a majority of patients have an improvement of the liver biochemistry after this therapy, 20% to 40% of patients have insufficient or no response to UDCA. Since 2016, obeticholic acid has been approved by the Food and Drug Administration and European Medicines Agency as a second-line treatment in association with UDCA in nonresponders to first-line therapy or in those intolerant to UDCA monotherapy. Moreover, several molecules targeting pathways involved in cholestasis or immune-related mechanisms might soon be available. It follows the importance of risk-stratification of patients' management based on the treatment response profile to allocate the best treatment to the right patient and improve the overall management.

Age and gender

Age and gender were shown to influence response to treatment with UDCA in PBC in the UK-PBC national cohort.[27] Gender was not confirmed, however, to be a predictor of treatment response in the international cohort of the Global PBC Study Group.[28]

Younger age at diagnosis was strongly and independently associated with response to UDCA, with an approximately linear relationship between age and the probability of response; rates ranged from 90% for patients greater than 70 years to 50% for those younger than age 30. The authors suggest that the relationship between age at diagnosis and likelihood of UDCA response was explicable by the effect of hormones, such that high estrogen levels increase resistance to effective treatment.[27] Furthermore, age and gender seemed to correlate with symptoms. Young girls were more likely to have fatigue and pruritus than older and male patients. The Newcastle group showed that fatigue is associated with a reduced survival.[29] Whether this translates in a worse outcome for young women is not clear.

Liver biochemistry

It is well established that the liver function tests (LFTs) on treatment with UDCA strongly predict LT-free survival in PBC.[30] This observation has prompted the development of several prognostic models based on the UDCA response that may be used to stratify patients according to their risk of developing chronic liver failure.

UDCA biochemical response can be assessed using either a qualitative definition based on binary variables or quantitative scoring systems computed from continuous parameters.[2] All these definitions and scores have been developed to be used only after 1 year of UDCA therapy to stratify according to treatment response.

Qualitative definitions Qualitative definitions use thresholds of the LFTs, such as bilirubin, transaminases, and ALP, after 6 months to 24 months of treatment with UDCA on a stable, optimized dose (13–15 mg/kg/d) to dichotomize patients into responders or nonresponders. The best-known of these binary definitions are reported in **Box 2**. Their accuracy in predicting death or LT has been validated externally[27] and they have all been proposed in the recent Clinical Practice Guidelines of EASL 2017.[2] Where binary

---

Box 2
Biochemical response criteria for risk stratification in ursodeoxycholic acid–treated primary biliary cholangitis patients and characteristics of the cohorts where they were developed

Response Definitions and Prognostic Models	Definition and Parameters Evaluated	Type of Prediction	Number of Patients	Centers
Paris I, 2008	ALP <3 × ULN, AST <2 × ULN and bilirubin ≤1 mg/dL after 1 y	Dichotomous	292	Single center
Barcelona, 2006	>40% decrease of ALP or normalization after 1 y	Dichotomous	192	Single center
Toronto, 2010	ALP ≤1.67 × ULN after 2 y	Dichotomous	69	Single center
Paris II, 2011	ALP ≤1.5 × ULN, AST ≤1.5 × ULN and bilirubin ≤l mg/dL after 1 y	Dichotomous	165	Single center
Rotterdam, 2009	Normalization of abnormal bilirubin and/or albumin after 1 y	Dichotomous	375	Single center
GLOBE score, 2015	Age, bilirubin, albumin, ALP, platelets	Continuous	2488	15 tertiary centers
UK-PBC score, 2016	Bilirubin, alanine aminotransferase (ALT)/AST ALP, platelets, albumin	Continuous	1916	155 secondary and tertiary centers

definitions are used for risk stratification, it is advised to use a definition with higher sensitivity but lower specificity. Possibly for this reason, the POISE trial definition of UDCA nonresponse (total bilirubin >1 × upper limit of normal [ULN] or ALP ≥1.67 × ULN) seems to have become the commercial standard, included in the eligibility criteria or endpoints of the phase I/II study of FFP104 by Fast Forward Pharmaceuticals (Utrecht, Netherlands); phase II study of LJN452 by Novartis (Basel, Switzerland); and phase II study of MBX-8025 by CymaBay (Newark, California, USA) Therapeutics (for details, see https://clinicaltrials.gov/). EASL advocates ALP less than 1.5 × ULN as the threshold at which long-term risk becomes clinically meaningful compared with a control healthy population.[2]

The main advantage of dichotomous definition is that they are easy to use. Such definitons do, however, have limitations because they could potentially lead to loss of important predictive information. Most importantly, they imply there are only 2 levels of risk, which is inaccurate. There is a continuous relationship between the individual LFT and the risk of liver death or LT.[31] Thus, dichotomous definitions fail to quantify intermediate levels of risk. Furthermore, they ignore the relationship between risk and time. They do not indicate whether the high-risk patient will need an LT tomorrow or 15 years in the future.

Quantitative scoring systems Proposed by the UK-PBC Research Group and the Global PBC Study Group,[28,31] quantitative scoring systems enable hepatologists to overcome the limitations of the binary risk stratification. In particular, these models quantify an individual's risk in relation to time. In comparison with the binary definition of response that only evaluate parameters of disease activity, they include surrogate markers of disease stage. Both UK-PBC and GLOBE outperform the Paris I definition.[32]

Each risk score includes the LFTs after treatment with UDCA as well as surrogate measurements of disease stage (see **Box 2**). In addition, the GLOBE score includes the age at diagnosis. In both risk scores, all the predictive variables are continuous—and treated as such. The UK-PBC risk score estimates the risk of LT or liver-related death occurring within 5 years, 10 years, or 15 years. The GLOBE score predicts LT-free survival at 3 years, 5 years, 10 years, and 15 years. Both risk scores were shown to outperform previous models, with C statistics at 15 years in the validation cohorts of 0.90 and 0.82, respectively.

In clinical practice, the UK-PBC and GLOBE scores should be most useful to identify patients who would obtain greatest benefit from further risk-reduction using second-line therapy. This is timely with several potential disease-modifying agents for PBC in phase II or III clinical trials. The UK-PBC and GLOBE scores may also be used to identify low-risk patients, for whom follow-up in primary care may be appropriate. There are no clear-cut thresholds that should prompt addition of second-line therapies or de-escalation of follow-up back to primary care. These thresholds vary from one patient to the next, influenced by the patient profile (age, fibrosis stage, and severity of itch, among others), side effects, and cost-effectiveness of a specific agent.

To date, metabolomics analysis of various classes of blood metabolites has been proposed only to define distinct profiles in patients with PBC. It would also allow, however, classifying patient responsiveness to therapies. The circulating metabolome capturing different metabolites classes (eg, BAs, aminoacids, acylcarnitines, Krebs cycle intermediates, lipids species, among the others), some of which in key biochemical pathways are known to be involved in PBC responsiveness, might be able to be defined by open (untargeted) and close (targeted) approaches. These might be integrated in the predicting model of treatment response to UDCA the authors recently proposed to develop enhanced predictive approaches for identification of high-risk patients earlier in the disease and facilitating application of enhanced therapy in a more timely fashion.[33]

Primary Biliary Cholangitis–Specific Autoantibody Profile

The anti-gp210 targets glycoprotein 210 of the nuclear pore complex. It is reportedly associated with more aggressive disease. In 3 studies from Italy and Japan, the presence of anti-gp210 antibodies was associated with more advanced disease, suggesting that anti-gp210 antibodies might be related to hepatocellular failure-type progression.[32] More recently, antibodies against hexokinase (HK1) and a nuclear protein involved in the metabolism of collagen (KL-p) have been shown sensitive and specific for detection of PBC and could be useful in diagnosis in Anti-mitochondrial M2 antibody (AMA-M2) negative, gp210 antibody negative, and sp100 antibody-negative patients. Furthermore, investigators found a correlation between the presence of antibodies anti-HK1 and disease progression, with lower transplant-free survival.[34] The PBC-specific antinuclear antibodies (ANAs) are still of limited validity in clinical practice because studies showing their prognostic role are limited and only retrospective. Longitudinal, large-scale studies using time-to-event data are needed to confirm their role as reliable markers of prognosis.

PERSPECTIVES OF PRECISION MEDICINE IN PRIMARY BILIARY CHOLANGITIS

To facilitate the identification of high-risk individuals for cost-effective disease monitoring and second-line therapies, mounting efforts have been put forth to develop risk prediction models, including biochemical variables with good accuracy and calibration regarding survival. The next step is the identification and incorporation of novel biomarkers, including genetic and molecular biomarkers, to allow identification of disease variants and trajectory, and to estimate the risk of disease progression and the likelihood of treatment response, paving the way for PM in PBC.

The PM initiative ongoing in PBC, as in many other fields of medicine, promises a new era of health care with targeted disease treatment and management. This features a longitudinal study of national and international cohorts of 1000 or more people with large quantity of data and biospecimens necessary to conduct a wide range of studies, with the aim of customizing interventions based on a person's profile.

Conducting a large study cohort study is challenging from several aspects: identification of financial resources needed for implementing such a large-scale project; time required to obtain meaningful results—this is a major problem in PBC due to its indolent nature, where prospective studies of outcomes would span decades to allow for a robust number of endpoints to occur; obtaining permission for data sharing and the need for researchers to recontact/consent participants; concerns about privacy, security, and access to individual data and health records; and coordination, transparency, and governance.

PM is expected to benefit from combining genetic and molecular studies with high-throughput methods, that is, genomics, transcriptomics, proteomics, and metabolomics, among others. These methods permit the determination of thousands of molecules within a tissue or biological fluid that can configure the signature of a disease. The use of these methods is demanding in terms of the design of the study, acquisition, storage, analysis, and interpretation of the data.

When carried out within the adequate medical context, genetic screens are powerful tools for identifying new genes and variations within genes that are involved in specific physiopathologic processes. An example in hepatology is the variant of patatin-like phospholipase domain-containing protein 3 gene (PNPLA3) that has been associated with the susceptibility and histologic severity of nonalcoholic fatty liver disease (NALFD).[35] PNPLA3 has been proposed as a novel biomarker for (gene-based) classification of NALFD and should be considered in the diagnostic work-up of this disease.

Genetic information will likely help advance the field of pharmacogenomics. Many single-nucleotide polymorphisms (SNPs) have been used to predict outcomes of specific pharmacologic agents. Some SNPs are used to predict whether an individual is susceptible to side effects from a certain class of drugs. Several groups, including the authors', are trying to create simpler tools that combine genetic and molecular data along with clinical and demographic parameters to predict treatment response to UDCA. In theory, this could be used at the outset to decide whether to escalate treatment of high-risk patients, offering second-line treatment at the outset.

An example of how genomics can be brought to real practice is the 100,000 Genomes Project, which was launched in 2012 in the United Kingdom. This project is performing whole-genome sequencing of 100,000 genomes from 70,000 individuals with rare diseases, their families, and patients with cancer. The main aim of this program is to set up a genomic medicine service for National Health Service patients with potential benefits in disease prevention, management, and treatment. It will also stimulate the development of diagnostics, devices, medicines, and treatments based on a new understanding of the genetic and molecular basis of disease. Finally, it will build partnerships between National Health Service, academia, and industry.

Genomic technologies have made feasible investigating the expression of thousands of genes, that is, transcriptomics, at a time using large sets of samples. The clinical application of transcriptomics profiling to reveal novel gene expression signatures is challenging in a complex disease like PBC for the following reasons. PBC might result from a large number of different genes and biological pathways and several phenotypes; therefore, large cohorts of well-characterized patients are necessary to obtain genomic signatures of clinical relevance. Also, pathogenic (that may be immune-related) and prognostic genes signatures (that may be related to fibrosis progression rather than severity of biliary inflammation) might contain a large number of genes and the prediction algorithms may be complex and not easy to transfer to routine clinical practice. Finally, there is the problem of false-positive tests inherent to all high-throughput techniques where large data sets are analyzed. That said, when used correctly, transcriptomics technologies may be translated into scoring systems that can reproducibly predict clinical outcomes. An example in hepatology is the development of a simple risk score classifier based on the expression of a small number of genes that can predict in a reproducible manner overall survival of patients after surgical resection for HCC.[36]

Another branch of omics-based technology is the high-throughput identification and quantification of small-sized molecules, that is, metabolomics. There is increased interest in understanding which metabolic differences between normal and diseased tissues can lead to the development of more selective and effective treatments. The main aim of metabolomics research is the discovery of specific metabolic profiles in serum, urine, feces, tissues, and other biological materials that are associated with disease features, response to specific treatments, or survival. Blood is the most commonly collected (as serum or plasma) and stored biological fluid in epidemiologic studies and has been the most often used sample in metabolomics analyses to date. Because blood components are under tight homeostatic regulation, the extent of variation in blood metabolite concentration is limited. Urine samples represent a good alternative to blood and have greater capture of exogenous compounds, such as microbiota, drugs, and diet, and urine composition can vary a lot, especially in disease states. A 24-hour collection is preferred over spot urine collection because it provides a complete picture of cumulative metabolite excretion over a 24-hour period. However, 24-hour samples are difficult to collect for epidemiologic studies.

The development of metabolomics-based diagnostic and prognostic tests has the same problems inherent to all high-throughput techniques, that is, the detection of true relationships between a group of metabolites and disease, minimizing the risk of false-positive associations. An additional complication in metabolomics, compared with other omics-based methods, is the preparation and storage of the samples, due to large differences in solubility and stability among metabolites. This is particularly important in relation to epidemiologic studies because samples regularly undergo freeze-thaw cycles that may unpredictably affect the analytical results. Metabolic profiling can run in either targeted or untargeted mode. Targeted profiling separates a limited number of specific metabolites of known identity and is a more hypothesis-driven approach. In PBC, such an approach might be focused on markers of BA physiology, inflammation, and fibrosis. Untargeted approaches are applied to capture metabolic classes that escape target analysis (eg, Krebs cycle intermediates, short-chain fatty acids, nucleotides). Untargeted analysis does not require an a priori hypothesis and can be used to discover novel metabolic associations and disease pathways. Data density is high, however, and because analysis is not optimized for specific metabolites, metabolite identification and quantification may be difficult. Several targeted attempts to identify a metabolomics signature are ongoing in PBC; these highlighted altered metabolic pathways associated with glucose, fatty acid, and amino acid metabolites.[37,38] Effort is required to associate the metabolomics profile with clinical features, such as disease subphenotypes, symptoms, disease course, treatment response, and survival.

Before initiating such studies, it is of primary importance to have a robust hypothesis, which dictates the entire omics workflow and greatly influences the study outcomes. The hypothesis dictates which technologies to choose from (eg, genomic and transcriptomic approaches to study the immunologic signature of the disease; metabolomics approaches on plasma and urine to study the cholestatic component; and proteomic approach to identify markers of the different patterns of fibrosis progression in PBC), the sample to study (eg, circulating cells vs infiltrating cells and whole blood cells vs peripheral blood mononuclear cells), and which approaches to use (eg, targeted vs untargeted metabolomics study) to carry on the study. As a next step, integration of omics data (transomics) is useful, complementary, and more informative than if single omics stood alone, despite being challenging.

Omics-based research to develop PM, however, requires more than just accumulating data. First of all, it is necessary to develop standard protocols that yield consistent results in different laboratories so that data can be built into a single repository. Another problem is the integration of all the data generated by omics-based screens (such as RNAs, proteins, metabolites, protein-protein interactions, protein-lipid interactions, protein-nucleic acid interactions, and so on). Finally, practical application will necessitate the creation of tools by which omics information can be filtered and made readily accessible to clinicians who will incorporate it into medical decision making at the point of care. A key component to advance PM from the academic setting to the point of care in the community is the incorporation of genetic and molecular databases directly into a universal electronic medical record (EMR) system. An effective EMR system prompts practitioners to follow certain diagnostic or treatment algorithms based on an individual's information and reference genomic/molecular datasets stored in the EMR.

PM, when fully realized, has great potential to change the way patients are managed with PBC today. Knowing the genetic and/or molecular variations linked to specific disease phenotype might influence the way disease is screened for drugs are selected and disease progression is surveyed. Ideally, all patients who enter a health care system in the future will have their DNA/molecular profile routinely sequenced and analyzed at admission and entered into a database to enhance patient care. The cost of obtaining, analyzing, storing, and integrating this information will have to be balanced with the potential overall savings to the health care system.

SUMMARY

In view of forthcoming availability of novel drugs that might have a positive impact on morbidity and mortality of patients with PBC and thanks to the rise of high-throughput omics technologies, the PBC field is now moving more quickly toward clinical translation to support PM. PM development has a great potential to change the standard of care in diagnostics, therapeutics, and clinical trials in this disease. In the future, a diagnostic work-up of PBC patients may include information on genetic variants and molecular signature that may define a particular subtype of disease and provide an estimate of treatment response and survival. To reach this point, specific interventions are needed, such as sequencing more genomes, creating bigger biobanks, and linking biological information to health data in EMR. This hopefully will help to shed light on the pathogenic mechanisms of this condition and translate knowledge into new therapies and care pathways.

REFERENCES

1. Collins FS, Varmus H. A new initiative on precision medicine. N Engl J Med 2015; 372(9):793–5.
2. Hirschfield GM, Beuers U, Corpechot C, et al. EASL clinical practice guidelines: the diagnosis and management of patients with primary biliary cholangitis. J Hepatol 2017;67(1):145–72.
3. Poupon R, Chazouilleres O, Corpechot C, et al. Development of autoimmune hepatitis in patients with typical primary biliary cirrhosis. Hepatology 2006;44(1):85–90.
4. Chazouillères O, Wendum D, Serfaty L, et al. Primary biliary cirrhosis-autoimmune hepatitis overlap syndrome: clinical features and response to therapy. Hepatology 1998;28(2):296–301.
5. European Association for the Study of the Liver. EASL clinical practice guidelines: autoimmune hepatitis. J Hepatol 2015;63(4):971–1004.
6. Millar B, Wong LL, Green K, et al. Autoimmune hepatitis patients with poor treatment response have a distinct liver transcriptome: implications for personalised therapy. J Hepatol 2017;66(1):S364.
7. Ercole A, Magnoni S, Vegliante G, et al. Current and emerging technologies for probing molecular signatures of traumatic brain injury. Front Neurol 2017;8:450.
8. Vleggaar FP, van Buuren HR, Zondervan PE, et al, Dutch Multicentre PBC Study Group the DMP Study. Jaundice in non-cirrhotic primary biliary cirrhosis: the premature ductopenic variant. Gut 2001;49(2):276–81.
9. Liberal R, Grant CR, Sakkas L, et al. Diagnostic and clinical significance of anti-centromere antibodies in primary biliary cirrhosis. Clin Res Hepatol Gastroenterol 2013;37(6):572–85.
10. Nakamura M, Kondo H, Tanaka A, et al. Autoantibody status and histological variables influence biochemical response to treatment and long-term outcomes in Japanese patients with primary biliary cirrhosis. Hepatol Res 2015;45(8):846–55.
11. Nakamura M, Kondo H, Mori T, et al. Anti-gp210 and anti-centromere antibodies are different risk factors for the progression of primary biliary cirrhosis. Hepatology 2007;45(1):118–27.
12. Navasa M, Parés A, Bruguera M, et al. Portal hypertension in primary biliary cirrhosis. J Hepatol 1987;5(3):292–8.
13. Kew MC, Varma RR, Dos Santos HA, et al. Portal hypertension in primary biliary cirrhosis. Gut 1971;12(10):830–4.

14. Corpechot C, Abenavoli L, Rabahi N, et al. Biochemical response to ursodeoxy-cholic acid and long-term prognosis in primary biliary cirrhosis. Hepatology 2008; 48(3):871–7.

15. Carbone M, Sharp SJ, Heneghan MA, et al. P1198: histological stage is relevant for risk-stratification in primary biliary cirrhosis. J Hepatol 2015;62:S805.

16. Garrido MC, Hubscher SG. Accuracy of staging in primary biliary cirrhosis. J Clin Pathol 1996;49(7):556–9. Available at: http://www.ncbi.nlm.nih.gov/pubmed/ 8813953. Accessed January 15, 2018.

17. Ludwig J, Dickson ER, McDonald GS. Staging of chronic nonsuppurative destructive cholangitis (syndrome of primary biliary cirrhosis). Virchows Arch A Pathol Anat Histol 1978;379(2):103–12. Available at: http://www.ncbi.nlm.nih. gov/pubmed/150690. Accessed January 15, 2018.

18. Nakanuma Y, Zen Y, Harada K, et al. Application of a new histological staging and grading system for primary biliary cirrhosis to liver biopsy specimens: interob-server agreement. Pathol Int 2010;60(3):167–74.

19. Desmet VJ. Histopathology of cholestasis. Verh Dtsch Ges Pathol 1995;79: 233–40. Available at: http://www.ncbi.nlm.nih.gov/pubmed/8600686. Accessed January 15, 2018.

20. Goldfischer S, Popper H, Sternlieb I. The significance of variations in the distribu-tion of copper in liver disease. Am J Pathol 1980;99(3):715–30. Available at: http://www.ncbi.nlm.nih.gov/pubmed/7386600. Accessed January 15, 2018.

21. Kumagi T, Guindi M, Fischer SE, et al. Baseline ductopenia and treatment response predict long-term histological progression in primary biliary cirrhosis. Am J Gastroenterol 2010;105(10):2186–94.

22. Corpechot C, Carrat F, Poujol-Robert A, et al. Noninvasive elastography-based assessment of liver fibrosis progression and prognosis in primary biliary cirrhosis. Hepatology 2012;56(1):198–208.

23. Trivedi PJ, Bruns T, Cheung A, et al. Optimising risk stratification in primary biliary cirrhosis: AST/platelet ratio index predicts outcome independent of ursodeoxy-cholic acid response. J Hepatol 2014;60(6):1249–58.

24. Mayo MJ, Parkes J, Adams-Huet B, et al. Prediction of clinical outcomes in pri-mary biliary cirrhosis by serum enhanced liver fibrosis assay. Hepatology 2008; 48(5):1549–57.

25. Lichtinghagen R, Pietsch D, Bantel H, et al. The Enhanced Liver Fibrosis (ELF) score: normal values, influence factors and proposed cut-off values. J Hepatol 2013;59(2):236–42.

26. Poupon R, Poupon R, Calmus Y, et al. Is ursodeoxycholic acid an effective treat-ment for primary biliary cirrhosis? Lancet 1987;329(8537):834–6.

27. Carbone M, Mells GF, Pells G, et al. Sex and age are determinants of the clinical phenotype of primary biliary cirrhosis and response to ursodeoxycholic acid. Gastroenterology 2013;144(3):560–9.e7.

28. Lammers WJ, Hirschfield GM, Corpechot C, et al. Development and validation of a scoring system to predict outcomes of patients with primary biliary cirrhosis receiving ursodeoxycholic acid therapy. Gastroenterology 2015; 149(7):1804–12.e4.

29. Jones DE, Al-Rifai A, Frith J, et al. The independent effects of fatigue and UDCA therapy on mortality in primary biliary cirrhosis: results of a 9year follow-up. J Hepatol 2010;53(5):911–7.

30. Leuschner U, Fischer H, Kurtz W, et al. Ursodeoxycholic acid in primary biliary cirrhosis: results of a controlled double-blind trial. Gastroenterology 1989;97(5):

1268–74. Available at: http://www.ncbi.nlm.nih.gov/pubmed/2551765. Accessed January 16, 2018.

31. Carbone M, Sharp SJ, Flack S, et al. The UK-PBC risk scores: derivation and validation of a scoring system for long-term prediction of end-stage liver disease in primary biliary cholangitis. Hepatology 2016;63(3):930–50.

32. Yang F, Yang Y, Wang Q, et al. The risk predictive values of UK-PBC and GLOBE scoring system in Chinese patients with primary biliary cholangitis: the additional effect of anti-gp210. Aliment Pharmacol Ther 2017;45(5):733–43.

33. Carbone M, Nardi A, Carpino G, et al. Pre-treatment risk stratification in primary biliary cholangitis: A predictive model to guide first-line combination therapy. 50(1):21–2.

34. Reig A, Garcia M, Shums Z, et al. The novel hexokinase 1 antibodies are useful for the diagnosis and associated with bad prognosis in primary biliary cholangitis. J Hepatol 2017;66(1):S355–6.

35. Sookoian S, Pirola CJ. Meta-analysis of the influence of I148M variant of patatin-like phospholipase domain containing 3 gene (PNPLA3) on the susceptibility and histological severity of nonalcoholic fatty liver disease. Hepatology 2011;53(6): 1883–94.

36. Nault J-C, De Reyniès A, Villanueva A, et al. A hepatocellular carcinoma 5-gene score associated with survival of patients after liver resection. Gastroenterology 2013;145(1):176–87.

37. Hao J, Yang T, Zhou Y, et al. Serum metabolomics analysis reveals a distinct metabolic profile of patients with primary biliary cholangitis. Sci Rep 2017;7(1):784.

38. Bell LN, Wulff J, Comerford M, et al. Serum metabolic signatures of primary biliary cirrhosis and primary sclerosing cholangitis. Liver Int 2015;35(1):263–74.

Personalized Medicine in Gynecologic Cancer
Fact or Fiction?

Logan Corey, MD[a],*, Ana Valente, MD[a,1], Katrina Wade, MD[b]

KEYWORDS

- Personalized medicine • Precision medicine • Targeted therapies
- Gynecologic malignancies

KEY POINTS

- Personalized medicine is an evolving concept that centers around treating cancers based on tumor molecular profiling rather than location of origin.
- Tumor molecular profiling has allowed for several driver mutations to be identified in gynecologic malignancies and subsequent targeted therapies to be created.
- With direct to consumer marketing, patient demand for personalized medicine is increasing.

INTRODUCTION TO PERSONALIZED MEDICINE

Personalized medicine, also known as "precision medicine," is the science of individualizing cancer care by treating tumors based on their genetic makeup rather than their location of origin.[1] Both gene expressional profiling and genome-wide sequencing have played significant roles in making this possible.[2] Knowing a tumor's molecular sequence has allowed for creation of targeted therapies. Examples of current successful oncologic therapies include BRAF inhibitors (vemurafenib) used in melanoma treatment, RET inhibitors (sorafenib) used in advanced renal and hepatocellular carcinomas, and epidermal growth factor receptor or anaplastic lymphoma kinase inhibitors used in non–small-cell lung cancer.[3]

In gynecologic oncology, the application of personalized medicine is still a work in progress. Genetic offenders or "driver mutations" have been identified in

This article was repurposed from Obstetrics and Gynecology Clinics of North America 46.1 (Gynecologic Cancer Care: Innovative Progress- Carolyn Y. Muller).

Disclosure Statement: The authors have nothing to disclose.

[a] Department of Obstetrics and Gynecology, Ochsner Clinic Foundation, 2700 Napoleon Avenue, New Orleans, LA 70115, USA; [b] Department of Gynecologic Oncology, Ochsner Clinic Foundation, 2700 Napoleon Avenue, New Orleans, LA 70115, USA

[1] Present address: 1520 Saint Mary Street, Unit D, New Orleans, LA 70130.

* Corresponding author. 209 North Dupre Street, New Orleans, LA 70118.

E-mail address: logan.corey@ochsner.org

ovarian cancer (BRCA mutations, NOTCH, P13 K, BRAS/MEK, FOX 1, p53), endometrial cancer (TP53, PTEN, P1K3CA, and KRAS) and cervical cancers (P1K3CA, TP53, RB1).[1] Therapies that target these molecules are being developed and are effective by various mechanisms, including interruption of tumor cell stroma, vasculature, and aberrant signaling mechanisms.[4] Several of these mutations and therapies and their use and challenges are discussed in this article, as we explore the intricacies of personalized medicine in gynecologic malignancy: is it fact or fiction?

DRIVER MUTATIONS

Oncogenic mutations belong to 1 of 2 groups of proteins: oncogenes or tumor suppressor genes. Mutations to oncogenes cause cancer growth, whereas mutations to tumor suppressor genes cause failure of inhibition of cell growth, and therefore indirectly lead to cancer. These oncogenic mutations are known as "driver mutations." Individual oncogenes also contain genetic alterations such as substitutions, insertions, deletions, rearrangements, and loss of heterozygosity. These "passenger mutations" are mutations that are commonly associated with driver mutations that do not themselves cause cancer. Interestingly, there is recent evidence proposed that passenger mutations in cumulative may not be benign bystanders within or around cancer genes and can be harmful to cancer cells.[5]

Identification of driver mutations is of interest because it stands to reason that if either type of driver mutations could be identified and countered, the cancer would be cured or slowed. Successes in such endeavors in other oncology subspecialties, for example, use of the Philadelphia mutation as a target and the use of imatinib in the treatment of chronic myelogenous leukemia, have encouraged expansion of this body of work into other fields including gynecology oncology.[6] Furthermore, the relatively recent capability of researchers to sequence entire cancer genomes in a cost-effective way has allowed for a rapid broadening of the search for driver mutations and the exploration of their utility as possible targets in cancer treatment. Strategies include prediction of function models, machine learning models, and models that are based on the difference in mutation frequencies between driver and passenger mutations.[7] Tumor suppressor genes are generally more difficult to identify as driver mutations than oncogenes. It is much simpler to insert an oncogene into a cell line and evaluate for cancer growth than it is to remove a tumor suppressor gene from a cell line and monitor for cancer growth (ie, knockout models). Occasionally, a single cancer will have multiple driver mutations. This is consistent with the suggestion that some common cancers are thought to require 5 to 7 rate-limiting events on the way to becoming cancerous.[8]

Other ways of identifying driver mutations involve looking for similar mutations in cancers that are present at increased frequency relative to the background genome. This was demonstrated in a large study by the Cancer Genome Atlas that examined more than 400 high-grade serous ovarian adenocarcinomas that used the previous method and found more than 96% of these tumors were characterized by p53 mutations. Additional mutations were identified by cross-referencing other databases. Multiple other mutations were found in most of the tumors along with the p53 mutations, including mutations in *BRAF* (N581S), *PIK3CA* (E545 K and H1047 R), *KRAS* (G12D), and *NRAS* (Q61 R).[8]

Isolating driver mutations in gynecologic cancer has proven difficult. This is most likely due to the complexity and ubiquitous nature of the pathways involved.

Multiple pathways are of intense interest at the moment and seem to play a role in development of other cancer types including breast, gastrointestinal, and lung cancers.

TUMOR HETEROGENEITY

Tumor heterogeneity is one of the greatest challenges in the era of personalized medicine. Although studies such as The Cancer Genome Atlas Project (TCGA) and the NCI-Match have helped in our understanding of the molecular basis of gynecologic cancers, they have also highlighted both intertumor and intratumor heterogeneity.[9,10] Intratumor heterogeneity is the concept that multiple biopsies of a single tumor may contain genetic variation and multiple subclonal populations. Studies have highlighted that such extreme molecular diversity can exist in solid tumor biopsies, even when they are collected from the same patient.[11] Whole genome and whole exosome studies have also highlighted genomic heterogeneity during transition from primary tumor to recurrence to metastasis.[12] This presents a unique challenge, especially in attempts to identify curative treatment for advanced disease.[13]

CURRENT TARGETED THERAPIES
Antiangiogenic Therapies

Angiogenesis, or the creation of new vascular supply, plays a key role in successful tumorigenesis. It is a process driven by vascular endothelial growth factor (VEGF). Overexpression of VEGF leads to increased blood supply and subsequent increase in delivery of nutrients and oxygen to tumor beds.[14] Antiangiogenesis therapies target and inhibit VEGF. Bevacizumab is the most studied antiangiogenic agent used in gynecologic cancer treatment.[1] It is a recombinant monoclonal antibody and is the only antiangiogenic therapy approved by the Food and Drug Administration (FDA).[15] Several clinical trials have investigated bevacizumab and demonstrated its efficacy in the treatment of ovarian cancer,[16,17] although overall survival benefit is seen only when bevacizumab is used in combination with standard cytotoxic chemo and then followed by bevacizumab maintenance.[18] In addition, the GOG240 has shown improved progression-free and overall survival when bevacizumab is added to standard chemotherapy in advanced or recurrent cervical cancer.[19]

Poly-ADP-Ribose Polymerase Inhibitors

Poly-ADP-ribose polymerase (PARP) inhibitors are agents that interfere with DNA damage repair. Typically, PARP repairs single-strand DNA breaks.[20] If single-strand DNA breaks are unable to be repaired due to PARP inhibition and accumulate, the DNA replication fork is stalled. In this situation, the cell must rely on double-strand break repair (via the homologous recombination [HR] pathway) to be able to survive, a mechanism that is notoriously absent in BRCA-mutated cells.[1,20] This leads to BRCA-deficient cells being incredibly vulnerable to PARP inhibitors and likewise confers their sensitivity to platinum as HR is required to repair platinum-induced intrastrand and interstrand DNA cross links. Several clinical studies have confirmed PARP inhibitors are effective,[21,22] and have shown significant increase in progression-free survival with their use.[23] Currently, 3 PARP inhibitors are FDA approved: olaparib, rucaparib, and niraparib. The study of PARP inhibitors is still currently under way and the future holds promise that they will not only be reserved for patients with BRCA mutations but may also be used in patients whose tumors have functional defects in other DNA repair proteins.[14]

PHOSPHATIDYL INOSITOL 3-KINASE/AKT/MAMMALIAN TARGET OF RAPAMYCIN/ PHOSPHATASE AND TENSIN HOMOLOG

The phosphatidyl inositol 3-kinase (PI3K)/AKT/mammalian target of rapamycin (mTOR) pathway plays a critical role in the malignant transformation of human tumors and their subsequent growth, proliferation, and metastasis, including ovarian cancers.[24] Characteristic of cell cycle control pathways, there is a normal balance to the activators and inhibitors within these complex pathways and the PI3K/AKT/ mTOR pathway is no different. These interactions are currently being studied for their theoretic druggable and targetable proteins. At the most basic level, the checks and balances are summarized as the following.

Activated PI3K leads to downstream effects to activate AKT. Then AKT can directly activate mTORC1 or indirectly through phosphorylating Tuberin, which inhibits TSC1/TSC2 complex, which itself is an inhibitor of mTORC1. Activated mTORC1 leads to downstream effects encoding ribosomal proteins, elongation factors, and other proteins required for transition from G1 phase to S phase of cell cycle. Phosphatase and tensin homolog (PTEN) has a role to play in this pathway as a tumor suppressor. PTEN is a negative regulator of the PI3K-dependent AKT signaling and acts as an antagonist of phosphorylation of PIP2 to PIP3.[25]

The understanding of this pathway lends to understanding the separation of targets into 4 main categories: mTOR inhibitors, PI3K inhibitors, dual mTOR/PI3K inhibitors, and AKT inhibitors. Many phase 1 and phase 2 trials are being undertaken with the modest success. A phase III trial by GOG 170-I showed higher response rate to temsirolimus in patients with tumors that exhibited mTOR activity than patients with tumors without mTOR activity. Unfortunately, there seems to be possibility for resistance to inhibitors of the PI3K/AKT/mTOR pathway. The mechanism is unknown but speculated to involve loss of negative feedback loops normally induced when the pathway is active. Proposed mechanisms for combating this is combining these inhibitors with other agents that inhibit at different points of the pathway (**Fig. 1**).[24]

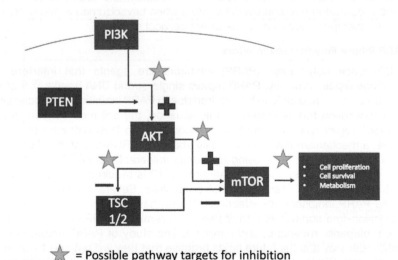

⭐ = Possible pathway targets for inhibition

Fig. 1. Simplified PI3K/AKT/mTOR pathway and possible points for inhibition.

Last, loss of function of PTEN has been detected in ovarian cancer as well as other cancers (eg, Cowden syndrome). This is of interest in PI3K/AKT/mTOR pathway because it is believed the ovarian cancer in PTEN knockout mouse models is caused through loss of inhibition of this pathway. Thus, inhibitors of PI3K/AKT/mTOR pathway may be beneficial as chemoprevention in selected patients with known PTEN mutations. It is especially hard to characterize the exact role of PTEN mutations in oncogenesis, as the protein acts in the cytoplasm as well as nucleus, and is also suspected to have antitumor effects by maintaining chromosomal stability, DNA double-strand break repair, and maintaining genome integrity.[26]

Consumer Marketing

The idea of personalized medicine began branching into the consumer market in the mid-2000s (DTC or Direct to Consumer). With the availability of high-throughput genomic sequencing, the price of testing an individual's genomic makeup reached a level affordable to the single consumer. Most of these tests are as simple as buccal or salivary swabs that are sent through the mail to the commercial laboratory. These private genetic laboratories offer testing for simple single-gene disorders (eg, cystic fibrosis) as well as pharmacogenomic tests to individualize drug treatment, including guidance for specific mutation-targeted treatment decisions for patients with cancers. They also include predictive genomic testing for complex disorders and traits such as hypertension and osteoporosis.[27] DTC marketing has become a popular among patients of all fields of medicine and the number of consumers of 23andMe and other similar DTC tests was more than 12 million in 2017. Most pertinent to our field, in March of 2018, the FDA authorized agencies to tell consumers whether they possess 1 of 3 germline mutations in the BRCA1 and BRCA2 genes.[28] **Table 1** lists just a few of the commercially available tumor sequencing assays.

Understanding and knowing BRCA1 and BRCA2 mutations, along with DNA mismatch repair genes of other hereditary cancer syndromes (eg, MLH1, MSH2,

Table 1
Examples of commercially available tumor gene sequencing tests

Tumor Test/Manufacturer	Targets Tested	Tissue	FDA Approval
FD1CDx	BRCA 1/2	Ovary	Yes
MSK-IMPACT	Varied, entire gene sequencing	Multiple	Yes[a]
SOLiD	Varied, entire gene sequencing	Multiple	Yes
Oncomine Dx Target Test	EGFR, BRAF, and ROS1	Lung	Yes
PathVysion	Her2/neu	Breast	Yes
PharmDx	Her2/neu	Breast	Yes
INFORM	Her2/neu	Breast	Yes
Dako	PD-L1	Lung	Yes
MI Profile	Many	Colon, lung	Yes
Solid Tumor Mutation Panel	Many	Multiple	Yes
SmartGenomics	Many	Multiple	Yes
Pervenio Lung NGS Assay	Many	Lung	Yes

Abbreviations: EGFR, epidermal growth factor receptor; FDA, Food and Drug Administration.
[a] Only at Sloan Kettering Memorial.

MSH6, and PMS2) presents significant opportunities in the treatment and prevention of some gynecologic cancers, including Lynch and Cowden, for example. This information can lead to alterations in screening and treatment plans. However, the availability of large population testing of these syndromes due to the DTC genetic testing leads to the idea that in general, the more genes tested, the more nonspecific the results, and the more variants of unknown significance will be found. Genetic counselors are a strained and poorly used source by the users of these genetic testing services. In one study, only 4% reported getting genetic counseling after receiving their genetic sequencing results, and 38% would have seen genetic counseling if one had been available. The risks of testing include increased anxiety or depression from positive results, uncertainty over inconclusive results, financial costs of testing, and difficulty navigating landscape of available testing modalities. Benefits of DTC genomic testing are narrow at this point, but by all accounts have a bright future. Current known benefits include more personalized prognosis, enhanced risk assessment, and improved triage to targeted therapies, such as using PARP inhibitors for BRCA carriers.

Treatment of gynecologic cancer with proprietary drugs, specific cancer therapies, and even specific hospital systems, is also affected by consumer directed advertisers. This is known as cancer related-direct to consumer advertisement (CR-DTCA).[29] CR-DTCA is particularly at risk for not clearly explaining costs, toxicity, and alternatives to patients as demonstrated in a retrospective review of warning letters sent by the FDA for not being fair and balanced, with the most (22%) being sent to CR-DTCA companies. Cancer therapy advertisement has the potential for wide-ranging affects including influencing treatment decisions and affecting the physician-patient relationship. In addition, gynecologic cancer presents challenges for clear information from advertisers to patients and oncologists, as within one general type of cancer (eg, ovarian cancer) there may be multiple potential targets, none of which seem to be singularly better than the other. This is in contrast to other cancers (eg, imatinib in patients with chronic myeloid leukemia with Philadelphia mutation) that have clear and successful treatment targets.

Overall, DTC affects oncologists as much or even more compared with other fields of medicine. Acceptance of the technology allowing for patient-obtained genetic information is necessary to help guide the conversation and inform patients and it would be "futile to try to reverse the course and reduce patients' access."[27] Personalized genetic sequencing tools currently have a role in BRCA and other DNA repair gene identification and can help with risk prediction as well as guide potential roles of chemoprevention. Expansion to more known genetic causes of gynecologic cancers, such as PTEN gene mutations and other homologous recombination-deficient genes, should be future goals of these sequencing tools.

The limiting factor in the usefulness of genetic sequencing tools seems to be with interpretation of the information for the consumers as well as the physicians. This is largely driven by lack of access to genetic counselors. Telemedicine, video chats, or requiring genetic counseling to be offered with the DTC genomic sequencing products may help increase access. Last, CR-DTCA seems to be more susceptible to bias information from marketers than other medical fields. The FDA is already monitoring advertisers but more scrutiny may be required in the future to ensure fair and balanced understanding of cancer therapies advertised to the general public.

PERSONALIZED TUMOR VACCINES

Personalized tumor vaccination is an aspect of treatment in gynecologic malignancies that has come in to play in recent years as we have gained knowledge that tumors may be largely immunogenic. Several studies have highlighted that host antitumor immune response plays a significant role in patient outcomes.[30,31] In ovarian cancer, the presence of tumor infiltrating lymphocytes (TILs) has been associated with increased progression-free survival and overall survival in patients with advanced disease.[30] Specifically, presence of CD-8 TILs has been found to correlate with survival in all stages and histologic types of ovary cancer.

Ovarian cancers are known to express tumor antigens that can serve as targets for peptide vaccination.[32] Peptide vaccinations are designed to target a variety of these antigens including NY-ESO-1, p53, WT-1, HER-2, and VEGF. They are often coadministered with GM-CSF to enhance immune response.[33,34] Whole tumor antigen vaccination is another option in personalized tumor vaccine development that provides for a wider range of tumor antigens.[35]

Dendritic cells (DCs) play a key role in development of cancer vaccination, as they serve as very potent antigen-presenting cells. We have seen in vitro that exposure of T cells to DCs pulsed with ovarian cancer antigens has resulted in the capability to kill autologous tumor cells.[36] Recently, a pilot clinical trial testing a personalized vaccine created by autologous DCs pulsed with oxidized autologous whole tumor lysate found personalized vaccination to induce T-cell response to autologous tumor antigen and increase survival.[37]

SUMMARY

In conclusion, personalized medicine in gynecologic oncology remains an evolving science. In recent years, the rapid advances in identification of the molecular drivers of gynecologic malignancies and the promise of targeted therapies have led to great enthusiasm. Although some of these therapies have been shown to have significant impact on outcomes (ie, PARP inhibitors in BRCA-mutated patients), others are still in need of additional research to identify when pathways may be most vulnerable to specific treatments (ie, PI3K in endometrial cancer). Tumor heterogeneity and tumor resistance contribute to the complexity of developing effective personalized therapies, as several studies have highlighted that tumor sampling may vary even among the same patient. We must continue to dedicate clinical research efforts to understanding how targeted therapies will be most applicable to patient care, especially as genetic testing becomes more available to patients through DTC markets.

REFERENCES

1. Barroilhet L, Matulonis U. The NCI-MATCH trial and precision medicine in gynecologic malignancy. Gynecol Oncol 2018;148(3):585–90.
2. Wiener C. Harrison's principles of internal medicine. New York: McGraw-Hill, Medical Pub. Division; 2008.
3. Coyne GO, Takebe N, Chen AP. Defining precision: the precision medicine initiative trials NCI-IMPACT and NCI-match. Curr Probl Cancer 2017;41(3):182–93.
4. Horwitz N, Matulonis U. New biologic agents for the treatment of gynecologic cancers. Hematol Oncol Clin North Am 2012;26:133–56.
5. McFarland CD, Korolev KS, Kryukov GV, et al. Impact of deleterious passenger mutations on cancer progression. Proc Natl Acad Sci U S A 2013;110(8):2910–5.
6. Druker BJ. Translation of the Philadelphia chromosome into therapy for CML. Blood 2008;112(13):4808–17.
7. Zhang J, Liu J, Sun J, et al. Identifying driver mutations from sequencing data of heterogeneous tumors in the era of personalized genome sequencing. Brief Bioinform 2014;15(2):244–55.

8. Michael S. The cancer genome. Nature 2009;458:719–24.
9. Getz G, Gabriel SB, Cibulskis K, et al. Integrated genomic characterization of endometrial carcinoma. Nature 2013;497(7447):67–73.
10. Integrated genomic analysis of ovarian carcinoma. Nature 2011;474(7573): 609–15.
11. Bashashati A, Ha G, Tone A. Distinct evolutionary trajectories of primary high-grade serous ovarian cancers revealed through spatial mutational profiling. J Pathol 2013;231(1):21–34.
12. Rodda E, Chapman J. Genomic insights in gynecologic cancer. Curr Probl Cancer 2017;41:8–36.
13. Testa U, Petrucci E, Pasquinin L, et al. Ovarian cancers: genetic abnormalities, tumor heterogeneity and progression, clonal evolution and cancer stem cells. Medicines (Basel) 2018;5(1) [pii:E16].
14. Berek J, Hacker N. Gynecologic oncology. 6th edition. Philadelphia: Lippincott Williams & Wilkins; 2014.
15. Liu J, Matulonis U. New strategies in ovarian cancer: translating the molecular complexity of ovarian cancer into treatment advances. Clin Cancer Res 2014; 20(20):5150–6.
16. Aghajanian C, Blank SV, Goff B, et al. OCEANS: a randomized, double blind, placebo-controlled phase III trial of chemotherapy with or without bevacizumab in patients with platinum sensitive recurrent epithelial ovarian, primary peritoneal or fallopian tube cancer. J Clin Oncol 2012;30(17):2039–45.
17. Pujade-Lauraine E, Hilpert F, Weber N, et al. Bevacizumab combined with chemotherapy for platinum resistant recurrent ovarian cancer: the AURELIA open-label randomized phase III trial. J Clin Oncol 2014;32(13):1302–8.
18. Coleman R, Brady M, Herzog T. Bevacizumab and paclitaxel-carboplatin chemotherapy and secondary cytoreduction in recurrent, platinum-sensitive ovarian cancer (MRG Oncology/Gynecologic Oncology Group study GOG-0213): a multicentre, open label randomized phase 3 trial. Lancet Oncol 2017;18(6):779–91.
19. Tewari K, Sill M, Long H, et al. Improved survival with bevacizumab in advanced cervical cancer. N Engl J Med 2014;370(8):734–43.
20. Liu J, Westin S. Rational selection of biomarker driver therapies for gynecologic cancers: the more we know, the more we know we don't know. Gyncol Oncol 2016;141:65–71.
21. Audeh M, Carmichael K, Penson R, et al. Oral poly(ADP-ribose) polymerase inhibitor olaparib in patients with BRCA 1 or BRCA2 mutations and recurrent ovarian cancer: a proof of concept trial. Lancet 2010;376(9737):245–51.
22. Coleman R, sill M, Bell K, et al. A phase II evaluation of the potent highly selective PARP inhibitor veliparib in the treatment of persistent or recurrent epithelial ovarian, fallopian tube or primary peritoneal cancer in patients who carry germline BRCA 1 or 2 mutation. An NRG Oncology/Gynecologic Oncology Group study. Gynecol Oncol 2015;137(3):386–91.
23. Oza AM, Cibula D, Oaknin A, et al. Olaparib plus paclitaxel and carboplatin (P/C) followed by olaparib maintenance treatment in patients (pts) with platinum-sensitive recurrent serous ovarian cancer (PSR SOC): a randomized, open-label phase II study [abstract]. J Clin Oncol 2012;30(Suppl):a5001.
24. Mabuchi S. The PI3K/AKT/mTOR pathway as a therapeutic target in ovarian cancer. Gynecol Oncol 2015;137(1):173–9.
25. Haddadi N, Lin Y, Travis G, et al. PTEN/PTENP1: 'regulating the regulator of the RTK-dependent PI3K/Akt signalling', new targets for cancer therapy. Mol Cancer 2018;17(1):37.

26. Patrinos GP, Baker DJ, Al-Mulla F, et al. Genetic tests obtainable through pharmacies: the good, the bad, and the ugly. Hum Genomics 2013;7(1):17.
27. Storrs C. Patients armed with their own genetic data raise tough questions. Health Aff 2018;37:690–3.
28. Schnipper LE, Abel GA. Direct-to-consumer drug advertising in oncology is not beneficial to patients or public health. JAMA Oncol 2016;2(11):1397–8.
29. Kim H. Trouble spots in online direct-to-consumer prescription drug promotion: a content analysis of FDA warning letters. Int J Health Policy Manag 2015;4(12): 813–21.
30. Zhang L, Conejo-Garcia JR, Katsaros D, et al. Intratumoral T cells, recurrence, and survival in epithelial ovarian cancer. N Engl J Med 2003;348:203–13.
31. Adams SF, Levine DA, Cadungog MG, et al. Intraepithelial T cells and tumor proliferation: impact on the benefit from surgical cytoreduction in advanced serous ovarian cancer. Cancer 2009;115:2891–902.
32. Chu CS, Kim SH, June CH, et al. Immunotherapy opportunities in ovarian cancer. Expert Rev Anticancer Ther 2008;8:243–57.
33. Mantia-Smaldone G, Corr B, Chu CS, et al. Immunotherapy in ovarian cancer. Hum Vaccin Immunother 2012;8(9):1179–91.
34. Odunsi K, Qian F, Matsuzaki J, et al. Vaccination with an NY-ESO-1 peptide of HLA class I/II specificities induces integrated humoral and T cell responses in ovarian cancer. Proc Natl Acad Sci U S A 2007;104:12837–42.
35. Chiang CL, Kandalaft LE, Coukos G. Adjuvants for enhancing the immunogenicity of whole tumor cell vaccines. Int Rev Immunol 2011;30:150–82.
36. Santin AD, Hermonat PL, Ravaggi A, et al. In vitro induction of tumor-specific human lymphocyte antigen class I-restricted CD8 cytotoxic T lymphocytes by ovarian tumor antigen-pulsed autologous dendritic cells from patients with advanced ovarian cancer. Am J Obstet Gynecol 2000;183:601–9.
37. Tanyi JL, Bobisse S, Ophir E, et al. Personal cancer vaccine effectively mobilizes antitumor T cell immunity in ovarian cancer. Sci Transl Med 2018;10(436) [pii: eaao5931].

Diffuse Large B-Cell Lymphoma and High-Grade B-Cell Lymphoma
Genetic Classification and Its Implications for Prognosis and Treatment

Jennifer L. Crombie, MD*, Philippe Armand, MD, PhD

KEYWORDS

- Diffuse large B-cell lymphoma • DLBCL • Cell of origin • Genomic classifications
- Targeted therapy • Precision medicine

KEY POINTS

- Diffuse large B-cell lymphoma (DLBCL) is a clinically and molecularly heterogeneous disease.
- Despite numerous robust prognostic biomarkers, predictive biomarkers are lacking.
- Attempts to use cell-of-origin classification for personalized therapy have thus far been unsuccessful.
- Recent advances in next-generation sequencing have advanced our understanding of the genomic heterogeneity of DLBCL.
- Prospective clinical trials are required to determine whether genomic-based classification of DLBCL can be used to guide treatment strategies.

INTRODUCTION

Diffuse large B-cell lymphoma (DLBCL) is the most common subtype of non-Hodgkin lymphoma, with approximately 27,000 new diagnoses in the United States each year.[1] DLBCL can occur de novo or as a result of transformation from a more indolent lymphoma. Although treatment with rituximab and multiagent chemotherapy results in cure for many patients, up to 40% of patients will have relapsed or refractory disease.[2]

This article was repurposed from Hematology/ Oncology Clinics of North America 33.4 (Non-Hodgkin Lymphoma- Caron A. Jacobson).
Disclosure Statement: J. Crombie has no conflicts of interest to disclose. P. Armand: Consultancy: Merck, BMS, Pfizer, Affimed, Adaptive, Infinity. Research funding (inst): Merck, BMS, Affimed, Adaptive, Roche, Tensha, Otsuka, Sigma-Tau
Medical Oncology, Harvard Medical School, Dana-Farber Cancer Institute, 450 Brookline Avenue, Boston, MA 02215, USA
* Corresponding author.
E-mail address: jennifer_crombie@dfci.harvard.edu

Surg Oncol Clin N Am 29 (2020) 115–125
https://doi.org/10.1016/j.soc.2019.08.009
1055-3207/20/© 2019 Elsevier Inc. All rights reserved.

Salvage chemotherapy followed by autologous stem cell transplantation remains the standard approach in this setting, yet fewer than half of patients will achieve long-term disease control.[3] Furthermore, patients who have refractory disease or relapse after transplant have limited therapeutic options with a poor overall survival.[4] Although chimeric antigen receptor T-cell therapy is a revolutionary treatment for patients with relapsed/refractory disease, still more than half of patients do not have a sustained response to treatment and are in urgent need of therapeutic options. [5]

Recently, comprehensive genomic analyses have allowed a better molecular characterization of DLBCL tumors, moving us closer toward the use of precision medicine in DLBCL. In this review, we highlight validated prognostic biomarkers as well as attempts made thus far to use them to personalize therapy in this heterogeneous disease. We also review the findings of more recent genomic analyses that could lead to a potential paradigm shift in management, possibly allowing for effective personalized therapy.

HETEROGENEITY OF DIFFUSE LARGE B-CELL LYMPHOMA

DLBCL has a clinically heterogeneous course, with approximately one-third of patients failing to respond durably to standard chemoimmunotherapy. This heterogeneity is thought to arise from the diverse origins of malignant lymphocytes, owing to antigen-exposed B cells transiting through the germinal center (**Fig. 1**). The germinal center is the site within a lymph node where B-lymphocytes, which have been exposed to antigens, undergo affinity maturation, developing the ability to produce high-affinity antibodies. Although this process is fundamental to immunologic function, it also involves mechanisms that predispose to malignant transformation. For

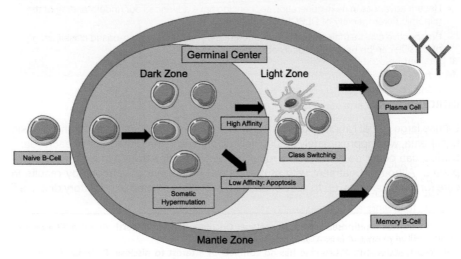

Fig. 1. B-cell development. This image represents the process of B-cell development within the germinal center of a lymph node. A naive B cell is exposed to an antigen before entering the germinal center. The B cell undergoes clonal expansion and somatic hypermutation in the process of affinity maturation. B cells that are able to make high-affinity antibodies will further undergo class switching before differentiating into a plasma cell or memory B cells. This process inherently leads to genomic instability that can promote lymphomagenesis. GCB-like DLBCL are thought to develop from B cells lacking markers of early postgerminal center cells, whereas ABC-like DLBCL display a transcriptional signature similar to cells before plasma cell differentiation.

example, high cellular proliferation rate, activation-induced cytidine deaminase-mediated immunoglobulin editing, and somatic hypermutation result in genomic instability, which can promote lymphomagenesis.[6,7] Genomic changes subsequently include multiple low-frequency genetic alterations including chromosomal translocations, somatic mutations, and copy-number alterations, which contribute to the high degree of molecular diversity seen in this disease and presumably lead to variable chemoresistance.[6,8]

VALIDATED PROGNOSTIC BIOMARKERS
International Prognostic Index

Currently a variety of prognostic factors are used to predict outcomes in DLBCL. The International Prognostic Index (IPI), which is based on 5 clinical characteristics, remains a mainstay of clinical risk stratification, highlighting disparities in outcomes in response to frontline therapy.[9,10] Clinical features comprising the IPI include age, lactate dehydrogenase, performance status, number of extranodal sites, and Ann Arbor stage. Whereas the IPI is a robust and accessible tool to effectively predict survival, it is unable to identify targetable vulnerabilities or guide the use of individualized therapy.

Cell-of-Origin Classification

Using gene expression profiling, molecularly distinct subtypes of DLBCL were identified in 2000, whose different genetic profile reflected different stages of B-cell development (see **Fig. 1**).[11,12] Germinal center B-cell (GCB)-like DLBCL expresses genes that define the germinal center B-cell signature and lack expression of early postgerminal center markers.[11,13] For example, recurrent *t(14;18)* translocations and amplification of the *c-rel* gene on chromosome 2p are found exclusively in this subtype of DLBCL.[12] The other main subtype of DLBCL is the activated B-cell (ABC)-like DLBCL, whose transcriptional signature resembles that of postgerminal center B cells blocked at plasmablastic differentiation. Recurrent trisomy 3, deletion of the *inhibitor of kinase 4A-alternative reading frame (INK4A/ARF)* locus and constitutive activation of the anti-apoptotic nuclear factor κB (NF-κB) signaling pathway are defining features of this subtype.[12,14,15] A smaller subset of tumors falls into a third group that does not express either set of genes at high levels. The cell-of-origin (COO) classification separates DLBCL tumors into the above 3 subtypes and has been repeatedly found to predict overall survival. Indeed, even with modern chemoimmunotherapy, patients with GCB subtype DLBCL often have superior outcomes following multiagent chemotherapy compared with patients with ABC-like DLBCL.[12] In 1 study, patients with GCB DLBCL had a 5-year survival of 60%, compared with 35% for those with ABC-like DLBCL following anthracycline-based chemotherapy.[12] Although the use of COO classification has become standard in clinical practice for prognostication, its prognostic validity has not been uniformly reproduced,[16] suggesting that potential residual heterogeneity within these subgroups may exist and carry important prognostic information. Furthermore, the difficulty of using standard immunohistochemistry markers to assign COO classification, which would facilitate the routine characterization of patients, has hampered the use of the COO classification for personalized therapy assignment.[17,18]

Comprehensive Clustering

An alternative transcriptional profiling classification, termed comprehensive consensus clustering (CCC), has also been used to subset distinct variants of

DLBCL.[19] This analysis identified 3 distinct groups: B-cell receptor, oxidative phosphorylation, and host response, highlighting the role of the tumor microenvironment and host inflammatory response as defining features in DLBCL. Although this study offered a nonoverlapping categorization from COO, and suggested potential rational therapeutic targets for each group, it has had a more limited role in clinical practice to date.

Double-Hit and Double-Expressor Status

Independently of the COO and CCC classifications, DLBCL molecular features involving the *MYC* oncogene have allowed the identification of a group of patients with aggressive clinical course. Specifically, within the GCB subtype, lymphomas with concurrent translocations involving *MYC* and *BCL-2* or *BCL-6*, termed double-hit lymphoma (DHL) or triple-hit lymphoma, have repeatedly been shown to have a particularly aggressive and refractory clinical course.[20,21] In the 2016 revision of the World Health Organization classification for lymphoma, a new entity, high-grade B-cell lymphoma with translocations involving *MYC* and *BCL-2* or *BCL-6*, was included, emphasizing the prognostic significance of these genomic aberrations. Even more recently, RNA sequencing data have also been used to define a gene expression signature that identifies GCB subtype DLBCL with a double-hit signature, even in the absence of *MYC* or *BCL-2* translocations, again identifying patients with a poorer prognosis.[22,23]

Efforts to use immunohistochemistry of MYC and BCL-2 to recapitulate the biology of DHL showed that combined increase in MYC and BCL-2 protein expression on the tumor cell surface, termed double-expressor lymphoma (DEL), is also an unfavorable subgroup with inferior outcomes after standard frontline therapy.[16,20] However, DEL and DHL are not identical or even strongly overlapping categorizations, and DEL status is not a surrogate of DHL status (or vice versa). Both DHL and DEL have also been associated with poor prognosis after autologous stem cell transplantation, with DHL and DEL associated with a reduction in progression-free survival (PFS) and DHL associated with a reduction in overall survival (OS).[24] Specifically, the 4-year PFS in patients with DEL compared with those with non-DEL was 48% versus 59% ($P = .049$) and the 4-year PFS in patients with DHL compared with those with non-DHL was 28% versus 57% ($P = .013$), and 4-year OS was 25% versus 61% ($P = .002$).[24] These data highlight that, although autologous stem cell transplantation remains a potentially curable option for patients with DLBCL, those with high-risk disease, such as those with DHL, are in need of novel treatment strategies both for frontline and for salvage treatment.

TRIALS TARGETING CELL-OF-ORIGIN SUBTYPES

Currently R-CHOP (rituximab, cyclophosphamide, doxorubicin, vincristine, and prednisone) remains the standard of care across most DLBCL subtypes in the frontline setting, although retrospective data suggest the value of more aggressive combination chemotherapy strategies in high-grade B-cell lymphoma with translocations involving *MYC* and *BCL-2* or *BCL-6*.[25–27] Despite the availability of numerous prognostic tools to predict therapy response, efforts to tailor therapeutic interventions for specific subtypes have so far been met with little success.

There have been numerous attempts to personalize therapy, especially across COO subtypes. Given the constitutive activation of NF-κB in ABC subtype DLBCL, which represents a high-risk subgroup of DLBCL, it has been hypothesized that inhibitors of NF-κB might sensitize cells to chemotherapy, thus improving outcomes.

Bortezomib is a proteasome inhibitor that blocks degradation of IκBα, consequently inhibiting NF-κB activity. Although there has been limited activity of bortezomib as a single agent in relapsed/refractory DLBCL, when combined with chemotherapy, a small study demonstrated that there were increased responses (83% vs 13%) and median OS (10.8 vs 3.4 months) in ABC compared with GCB DLBCL, respectively.[28] Although these data were encouraging, it should be noted that this study consisted of only 12 patients with ABC and 15 patients with GCB subtype DLBCL, and that the classification of COO used both gene expression profiling and the less-reliable method of immunohistochemistry.[28] Bortezomib was also tested in combination with R-CHOP for initial therapy for DLBCL, in which, unlike previous studies of R-CHOP alone, patients with GCB and ABC subtype DLBCL were found to have similar outcomes, suggesting potential selective improvement of outcome in ABC patients.[29] Based on these encouraging preliminary studies, a randomized phase 2 trial was developed comparing R-CHOP with R-CHOP plus bortezomib in patients with non-GCB subtype DLBCL as determined by immunohistochemistry.[30] Overall response rates with R-CHOP and R-CHOP plus bortezomib were 98% and 96%, respectively, and there was no significant OS with the addition of bortezomib.

Similar findings were seen with ibrutinib, an inhibitor of Bruton's tyrosine kinase (BTK). As ABC subtype DLBCL carry mutations that result in chronic active B-cell receptor signaling, ibrutinib was also theorized to have increased activity in this subtype. Although the phase 1/2 trial of ibrutinib monotherapy in relapsed/refractory DLBCL resulted in partial responses in 37% (14/38) of patients with ABC DLBCL, but in only 5% (1/20) of subjects with GCB DLBCL ($P = .0106$), confirmatory studies in the frontline setting have failed to demonstrate a benefit of adding ibrutinib to chemotherapy.[31] For example, a global, randomized, phase 3 trial of R-CHOP versus R-CHOP plus ibrutinib in patients with non-GCB DLBCL demonstrated no improvement in event-free survival with the addition of ibrutinib.[32] Similar studies with the addition of lenalidomide to frontline chemotherapy have also been performed, although phase 3 confirmatory studies are ongoing.[33–36]

GENOMIC UNDERPINNINGS OF DIFFUSE LARGE B-CELL LYMPHOMA

Growing evidence suggests that the failure of biomarkers such as COO to guide therapy stems from heterogeneity within traditional classification structures. More recently, techniques incorporating next-generation sequencing have exposed a more complex genomic variability in DLBCL. Such analyses have also identified a broad range of genomic aberrations that are potentially driving or contributing to lymphomagenesis.

Initial genomic analyses identified the genetic diversity of DLBCL, although they were limited by small sample size and limited scope.[37–39] One study, for example, identified frequent mutations in histone-modifying genes such as *MLL2*, which encodes a methyltransferase enzyme, and MEF2B, a calcium-regulated gene that cooperates with CREBBP and EP300 in acetylating histones.[37] In a subsequent study, whole-exome sequencing revealed recurrent mutations in genes known to be functionally relevant in DLBCL, including *MYD88*, *CARD11*, *EZH2*, and *CREBBP*, as well as in a variety of genes with unknown significance.[39] In addition to mutations, copy-number alterations are also common in DLBCL. In 1 small analysis of DLBCL samples, 90 copy-number alterations were identified across 6 individuals studied, with significant variability across samples.[38] Another analysis of a larger cohort of patients identified 47 recurrent copy-number alterations, including 21 copy gains and 26 copy losses, with frequencies of 4% to 27%, many of which resulted in decreased p53 activity and perturbed cell-cycle regulation.[8] Although these studies were fundamental to the recognition of the genomic complexity of DLBCL, given the small numbers of patients studied, they failed to identify a framework to categorize patients or guide the use of therapy.

More recently, larger-scale whole-exome sequencing and transcriptome analyses from a cohort of more than 1000 patients with DLBCL has comprehensively identified single-nucleotide variants, insertions/deletions (indels), and copy-number alterations in DLBCL, resulting in the discovery of approximately 150 recurrently mutated driver genes, including some that occur at low frequency and would be missed in smaller studies.[40] Although most identified mutations occurred in GCB and ABC subtypes, a small number of alterations were specific to each COO classification. For example, *EZH2*, *SGK1*, *GNA13*, *SOCS1*, *STAT6*, and *TNFRSF14* mutations were more frequently mutated in GCB DLBCLs, whereas *ETV6*, *MYD88*, *PIM1*, and *TBL1XR1* were more frequently mutated in ABC DLBCLs.[40] The functional roles of these mutations were also analyzed by unbiased CRISPR screens, identifying a much smaller subset of genes with functional relevance.

Additional studies have since been performed, incorporating analyses of a broad range of genomic aberrations in large cohorts of patients with DLBCL. In 1 study of 151 patients, a total of 761 potential driver mutations were identified and all tumors were found to have copy-number alterations, including frequent losses, gains, and amplifications.[41] The authors also analyzed the clinical influence of genetic alterations in predefined functional pathways. For example, mutations in the NOTCH signaling pathway and in *TP53/CDKN2A* were associated with poorer outcomes, whereas JAK/STAT pathway mutations were associated with improved outcomes.[41] They also found that 46% of patients had at least 1 genomic alteration that could be a predictive biomarker of drug response in DLBCL or other lymphomas and could potentially be exploited to guide targeted therapy. [41]

A similar study incorporated whole-exome and transcriptome sequencing, array-based copy-number analysis, and targeted amplicon resequencing in 574 DLBCL samples.[42] This study specifically investigated how such genetic aberrations could refine the categories of ABC or GCB subtypes. *CD79B* and *MYD88*[L265P] mutations were enriched in ABC subtype DLBCLs, and *EZH2* mutations and *BCL-2* translocations were frequently found in the same tumor and were much more frequent in GCB tumors. Mutations such as *NOTCH2* and *BCL-6* fusions were less likely to be classifiable by COO. The authors used these finding to classify DLBCL tumors into 4 genomic subtypes, characterized by (1) *CD79B/MYD88*[L265P] double mutations, (2) *NOTCH2* mutations or *BCL6* fusions in ABC or unclassified DLBCL, (3) *NOTCH1* mutations, and (4) *EZH2* mutations or *BCL2* translocations.[42] These subtypes had prognostic relevance even after accounting for COO assignment, with inferior responses found in patients with *CD79BMYD88*[L265P] double mutations and *NOTCH1* mutations.[42] Of note, these genomic subtypes comprised just under half of the cases studied, suggesting that a distinct pattern of genomic heterogeneity might be identified in the remaining group of patients.

An additional analysis of a large of cohort of previously untreated patients with DLBCL identified distinct genomic subtypes of DLBCL using comprehensive genomic analyses.[6] Recurrent mutations, somatic copy-number alterations, and structural variants were used to characterize patient samples into distinct genomic clusters using nonnegative matrix factorization classification (**Table 1**), and genomic signatures subsequently correlated with outcome data. Interestingly, this genomic-based classification suggested heterogeneity even within the COO subgroups, with a newly identified poor-risk GCB subtype and a favorable-risk ABC subtype. Specific subsets of tumors

Table 1
Newly identified genomic clusters of DLBCL

	Cluster 1	Cluster 2	Cluster 3	Cluster 4	Cluster 5
Characteristic mutations	BCL-6 structural variants with mutations in NOTCH2 signaling pathway components	Biallelic inactivation of TP53, 17p copy loss, 9p21.3/CDKN2A copy loss and associated genomic instability	BCL2 structural variants, inactivating mutations and/or copy loss of PTEN and alterations of epigenetic enzymes	Alterations in JAK/STAT and BRAF pathway components and multiple histones	Near-uniform BCL2 copy gain, frequent activating MYD88^{L265P}, CD79B mutations
Cell of origin	ABC	COO independent	GCB	GCB	ABC
Risk	Low-risk		High-risk	Low-risk	High-risk
Other features	Features of extrafollicular, possibly marginal zone, lymphoma				Extranodal tropism

Data from Chapuy B. Stewart C, Dunford AJ, et al. Molecular subtypes of diffuse large B cell lymphoma are associated with distinct pathogenic mechanisms and outcomes. Nat Med 2018;24(5):679–90.

(clusters) with discrete genetic signatures included: (1) high-risk ABC DLBCLs with near-uniform *BCL2* copy gain, frequent activating *MYD88*[L265P], *CD79B* mutations, and extranodal tropism (cluster 5); (2) low-risk ABC DLBCLs with genetic features of an extrafollicular, possibly marginal zone, origin (cluster 1); (3) high-risk GCB DLBCLs with *BCL2* structural variants, inactivating mutations and/or copy loss of *PTEN* and alterations of epigenetic enzymes (cluster 3); (4) a newly defined group of low-risk GCB DLBCLs with distinct alterations in JAK/STAT and BRAF pathway components and multiple histones (cluster 4); and (5) an ABC/GCB-independent group of tumors with biallelic inactivation of *TP53*, 9p21.3/*CDKN2A* copy loss and associated genomic instability (cluster 2). The genetically distinct subtypes were found to have significant differences in PFS, with a significantly higher risk of relapse in cluster 5 ABC DLBCL and cluster 3 GCB DLBCL.

These recent comprehensive genomic analyses have shed light on the previously unappreciated genomic complexity of DLBCL, the limitations of gene expression-based classification systems, and the challenge of adopting a uniform treatment approach in this disease. They also suggest specific therapeutic approaches to genomically characterized subsets. For example, although ibrutinib did not improve outcomes when added to chemotherapy for patients with non-GCB DLBCL, there may be a role for BTK inhibition in distinct genomic subtypes of DLBCL, such as in patients with *CD79B/MYD88*[L265P] double mutations[42] or those within the high-risk ABC DLBCLs, with near-uniform *BCL2* copy gain, and frequently activating *MYD88*[L265P] and *CD79B* mutations, as recently described (cluster 5).[6,42] Similarly, there may be a role for other targeted therapies, including EZH2, PI3K, and BCL-2 inhibitors in distinct genomic subtypes of DLBCL. In fact, preclinical work has already identified preferential activity of targeted therapies in individual genomic subtypes of DLBCL that may have clinical implications.[43] Prospective clinical trials are required to validate the use of genomic classifications and to determine whether they can be used to guide the use of targeted therapy.

USE OF GENOMIC INFORMATION IN PATIENTS

Although major progress has been made in understanding the genomic landscape of DLBCL, this understanding has not yet translated into clinical success. Some of the limitations of using comprehensive genomic analyses for therapy selection include the high cost, long turn-around times, and necessary access to sophisticated sequencing platforms that are typically restricted to research centers. Further distillation of genomic data into more limited and more broadly useable sequencing panels will likely be necessary for the short-term deployment of genomically driven treatment strategies. In addition, continued investigation of the role of liquid biopsies, in which tumor DNA from the peripheral blood serves as a surrogate for tumor biopsies, may improve the availability of genomic information and provide a means to track genomic changes with time.[44] Overall, the expansion of genomic data and more sophisticated classification methods currently under development hold great promise to transform the treatment approach to this disease and to improve the outcomes for those with high-risk disease.

REFERENCES

1. Teras LR, DeSantis CE, Cerhan JR, et al. 2016 US lymphoid malignancy statistics by World Health Organization subtypes. CA Cancer J Clin 2016;66(6):443–59.
2. Sehn LH, Donaldson J, Chhanabhai M, et al. Introduction of combined CHOP plus rituximab therapy dramatically improved outcome of diffuse large B-cell lymphoma in British Columbia. J Clin Oncol 2005;23(22):5027–33.

3. Philip T, Guglielmi C, Hagenbeek A, et al. Autologous bone marrow transplantation as compared with salvage chemotherapy in relapses of chemotherapy-sensitive non-Hodgkin's lymphoma. N Engl J Med 1995;333(23):1540–5.
4. Crump M, Neelapu SS, Farooq U, et al. Outcomes in refractory diffuse large B-cell lymphoma: results from the international SCHOLAR-1 study. Blood 2017; 130(16):1800–8.
5. Neelapu SS, Locke FL, Bartlett NL, et al. Axicabtagene ciloleucel CAR T-cell therapy in refractory large B-cell lymphoma. N Engl J Med 2017;377(26):2531–44.
6. Chapuy B, Stewart C, Dunford AJ, et al. Molecular subtypes of diffuse large B cell lymphoma are associated with distinct pathogenic mechanisms and outcomes. Nat Med 2018;24(5):679–90.
7. Basso K, Dalla-Favera R. Germinal centres and B cell lymphomagenesis. Nat Rev Immunol 2015;15(3):172–84.
8. Monti S, Chapuy B, Takeyama K, et al. Integrative analysis reveals an outcome-associated and targetable pattern of p53 and cell cycle deregulation in diffuse large B cell lymphoma. Cancer Cell 2012;22(3):359–72.
9. International Non-Hodgkin's Lymphoma Prognostic Factors Project. A predictive model for aggressive non-Hodgkin's lymphoma. N Engl J Med 1993;329(14): 987–94.
10. Ziepert M, Hasenclever D, Kuhnt E, et al. Standard International prognostic index remains a valid predictor of outcome for patients with aggressive CD20+ B-cell lymphoma in the rituximab era. J Clin Oncol 2010;28(14):2373–80.
11. Alizadeh AA, Eisen MB, Davis RE, et al. Distinct types of diffuse large B-cell lymphoma identified by gene expression profiling. Nature 2000;403(6769):503–11.
12. Rosenwald A, Wright G, Chan WC, et al. The use of molecular profiling to predict survival after chemotherapy for diffuse large-B-cell lymphoma. N Engl J Med 2002;346(25):1937–47.
13. Pasqualucci L, Dalla-Favera R. Genetics of diffuse large B-cell lymphoma. Blood 2018;131(21):2307–19.
14. Bea S, Zettl A, Wright G, et al. Diffuse large B-cell lymphoma subgroups have distinct genetic profiles that influence tumor biology and improve gene-expression-based survival prediction. Blood 2005;106(9):3183–90.
15. Lenz G, Wright G, Dave SS, et al. Stromal gene signatures in large-B-cell lymphomas. N Engl J Med 2008;359(22):2313–23.
16. Staiger AM, Ziepert M, Horn H, et al. Clinical impact of the cell-of-origin classification and the MYC/BCL2 dual expresser status in diffuse large B-cell lymphoma treated within prospective clinical trials of the German High-Grade Non-Hodgkin's Lymphoma Study Group. J Clin Oncol 2017;35(22):2515–26.
17. Hans CP, Weisenburger DD, Greiner TC, et al. Confirmation of the molecular classification of diffuse large B-cell lymphoma by immunohistochemistry using a tissue microarray. Blood 2004;103(1):275–82.
18. Meyer PN, Fu K, Greiner TC, et al. Immunohistochemical methods for predicting cell of origin and survival in patients with diffuse large B-cell lymphoma treated with rituximab. J Clin Oncol 2011;29(2):200–7.
19. Monti S, Savage KJ, Kutok JL, et al. Molecular profiling of diffuse large B-cell lymphoma identifies robust subtypes including one characterized by host inflammatory response. Blood 2005;105(5):1851–61.
20. Green TM, Young KH, Visco C, et al. Immunohistochemical double-hit score is a strong predictor of outcome in patients with diffuse large B-cell lymphoma treated with rituximab plus cyclophosphamide, doxorubicin, vincristine, and prednisone. J Clin Oncol 2012;30(28):3460–7.

21. Johnson NA, Savage KJ, Ludkovski O, et al. Lymphomas with concurrent BCL2 and MYC translocations: the critical factors associated with survival. Blood 2009;114(11):2273–9.
22. Ennishi D, Jiang A, Boyle M, et al. Double-hit gene expression signature defines a distinct subgroup of germinal center B-cell-like diffuse large B-cell lymphoma. J Clin Oncol 2019;37(3):190–201.
23. Sha C, Barrans S, Cucco F, et al. Molecular high-grade B-cell lymphoma: defining a poor-risk group that requires different approaches to therapy. J Clin Oncol 2019;37(3):202–12.
24. Herrera AF, Mei M, Low L, et al. Relapsed or refractory double-expressor and double-hit lymphomas have inferior progression-free survival after autologous stem-cell transplantation. J Clin Oncol 2017;35(1):24–31.
25. Wilson W, sin-Ho J, Pitcher B, et al. Phase III randomized study of R-CHOP versus DA-EPOCH-R and molecular analysis of untreated diffuse large B-cell lymphoma: CALGB/alliance 50303. Blood 2016;128:469.
26. Oki Y, Noorani M, Lin P, et al. Double hit lymphoma: the MD Anderson Cancer Center clinical experience. Br J Haematol 2014;166(6):891–901.
27. Petrich AM, Gandhi M, Jovanovic B, et al. Impact of induction regimen and stem cell transplantation on outcomes in double-hit lymphoma: a multicenter retrospective analysis. Blood 2014;124(15):2354–61.
28. Dunleavy K, Pittaluga S, Czuczman MS, et al. Differential efficacy of bortezomib plus chemotherapy within molecular subtypes of diffuse large B-cell lymphoma. Blood 2009;113(24):6069–76.
29. Ruan J, Martin P, Furman RR, et al. Bortezomib plus CHOP-rituximab for previously untreated diffuse large B-cell lymphoma and mantle cell lymphoma. J Clin Oncol 2011;29(6):690–7.
30. Leonard JP, Kolibaba KS, Reeves JA, et al. Randomized phase II study of R-CHOP with or without bortezomib in previously untreated patients with non-germinal center B-cell-like diffuse large B-cell lymphoma. J Clin Oncol 2017; 35(31):3538–46.
31. Wilson WH, Young RM, Schmitz R, et al. Targeting B cell receptor signaling with ibrutinib in diffuse large B cell lymphoma. Nat Med 2015;21(8):922–6.
32. Younes A, Sehn LH, Johnson P, et al. Randomized Phase III Trial of Ibrutinib and Rituximab Plus Cyclophosphamide, Doxorubicin, Vincristine, and Prednisone in Non-Germinal Center B-Cell Diffuse Large B-Cell Lymphoma. J Clin Oncol 2019. [Epub ahead of print].
33. Castellino A, Chiappella A, LaPlant BR, et al. Lenalidomide plus R-CHOP21 in newly diagnosed diffuse large B-cell lymphoma (DLBCL): long-term follow-up results from a combined analysis from two phase 2 trials. Blood Cancer J 2018; 8(11):108.
34. Nowakowski GS, LaPlant B, Macon WR, et al. Lenalidomide combined with R-CHOP overcomes negative prognostic impact of non-germinal center B-cell phenotype in newly diagnosed diffuse large B-cell lymphoma: a phase II study. J Clin Oncol 2015;33(3):251–7.
35. Nowakowski GS, Chiappella A, Witzig TE, et al. ROBUST: lenalidomide-R-CHOP versus placebo-R-CHOP in previously untreated ABC-type diffuse large B-cell lymphoma. Future Oncol 2016;12(13):1553–63.
36. King RL, Nowakowski GS, Witzig TE, et al. Rapid, real time pathology review for ECOG/ACRIN 1412: a novel and successful paradigm for future lymphoma clinical trials in the precision medicine era. Blood Cancer J 2018;8(3):27.

37. Morin RD, Mendez-Lago M, Mungall AJ, et al. Frequent mutation of histone-modifying genes in non-Hodgkin lymphoma. Nature 2011;476(7360):298–303.
38. Pasqualucci L, Trifonov V, Fabbri G, et al. Analysis of the coding genome of diffuse large B-cell lymphoma. Nat Genet 2011;43(9):830–7.
39. Lohr JG, Stojanov P, Lawrence MS, et al. Discovery and prioritization of somatic mutations in diffuse large B-cell lymphoma (DLBCL) by whole-exome sequencing. Proc Natl Acad Sci U S A 2012;109(10):3879–84.
40. Reddy A, Zhang J, Davis NS, et al. Genetic and functional drivers of diffuse large B cell lymphoma. Cell 2017;171(2):481–94.e15.
41. Karube K, Enjuanes A, Dlouhy I, et al. Integrating genomic alterations in diffuse large B-cell lymphoma identifies new relevant pathways and potential therapeutic targets. Leukemia 2018;32(3):675–84.
42. Schmitz R, Wright GW, Huang DW, et al. Genetics and pathogenesis of diffuse large B-cell lymphoma. N Engl J Med 2018;378(15):1396–407.
43. Bojarczuk K, Wienand K, Ryan JA, et al. Targeted inhibition of PI3Kalpha/delta is synergistic with BCL-2 blockade in genetically defined subtypes of DLBCL. Blood 2019;133(1):70–80.
44. Scherer F, Kurtz DM, Newman AM, et al. Distinct biological subtypes and patterns of genome evolution in lymphoma revealed by circulating tumor DNA. Sci Transl Med 2016;8(364):364ra155.

Oral Cancer

Genetics and the Role of Precision Medicine

Chia-Cheng Li, DDS, DMSc[a],*, Zhen Shen, PhD[b], Roxanne Bavarian, DMD[b,c],
Fan Yang, DDS, PhD[b], Aditi Bhattacharya, BDS, MDS, PhD[d]

KEYWORDS

- Oral cancer • Oral squamous cell carcinoma • Malignant transformation
- Epigenetics • Omics technology • Big data • Personalized medicine
- Precision medicine

KEY POINTS

- Oral squamous cell carcinoma (OSCC), a distinct subtype of head and neck squamous cell carcinoma, is typically human papillomavirus-negative and harbors *TP53* loss-of-function mutations.
- OSCC is thought to begin with cancer initiating cells that are able to self-renew and generate heterogeneous clones of neoplastic cells to comprise the tumor (ie, tumor heterogeneity).
- Carcinogenesis is a multistep process, which involves an accumulation of both genetic and epigenetic alterations in oncogenes and/or tumor suppressor genes.
- Metastasis is one of the major prognostic indicators in OSCC. Both epithelial-to-mesenchymal transition and interactions between OSCC cells and the tumor microenvironment play significant roles in this complex process.
- The integration of omics technologies, bioinformatics, and molecular biology uncovers complex, clinically meaningful information that greatly improves our understanding of the disease process.

INTRODUCTION TO ORAL CANCER

Cancer is a major global health issue. According to the GLOBOCAN project of the International Agency for Research on Cancer, there were approximately 14.1 million newly

This article was repurposed from Dental Clinics of North America 62.1 (Oral Cancer- Eric T. Stoopler and Thomas P. Sollecito).
[a] Department of Oral Medicine, Infection and Immunity, Harvard School of Dental Medicine, 188 Longwood Avenue, Boston, MA 02115, USA; [b] Harvard School of Dental Medicine, 188 Longwood Avenue, Boston, MA 02115, USA; [c] Division of Oral Medicine and Dentistry, Brigham and Women's Hospital, Francis Street, Boston, MA 02115, USA; [d] Department of Oral and Maxillofacial Surgery, NYU College of Dentistry, East 24th Street, New York, NY 10010, USA
* Corresponding author.
E-mail address: Chia-Cheng_Li@hsdm.harvard.edu

diagnosed cancer cases with 8.2 million deaths worldwide in 2012.[1] Globally, oral cancer is one of the leading cancers, accounting for 2% of all cancer cases, with a nearly 50% mortality rate.[1] Internationally, the highest rates of oral cancer are seen in South Asian countries, such as Sri Lanka, India, and Taiwan, which are attributed to the high rates of cigarette smoking and areca nut use in these countries.[2] In the United States, 48,330 cases of oral and oropharyngeal cancer are diagnosed each year, comprising approximately 3% of all cancer cases.[3–8] It is the eighth leading cancer in men, with more than two-thirds of oral cancer cases occurring in male patients.[1,3]

Multiple factors contribute to the initiation of oral cancer. In addition to the well-established roles of tobacco, alcohol, and areca nut as risk factors for oral cancer, high-risk human papillomavirus infection (eg, HPV-16 and HPV-18) has been identified as a significant risk factor for oropharyngeal cancer.[9] Recent studies over the past decade have revealed an increasing incidence of HPV-positive oropharyngeal cancer in developed countries, which exhibits a better prognosis than HPV-negative oral cancer.[10,11] Specific germline mutations are also associated with a higher incidence of oral cancer. For example, patients with Li-Fraumeni syndrome (germline *TP53* mutation) are predisposed to early-onset oral cancer.[12] Additionally, patients with Fanconi anemia, a condition characterized by defects in the DNA repair process and consequent chromosomal instability, are associated with aggressive oral cancers that present at a young age.[13,14] Due to defective telomerase maintenance, patients with dyskeratosis congenita exhibit a thousand-fold increased risk for developing oral cancer.[15]

Squamous cell carcinoma (SCC) constitutes more than 90% of all cancer cases arising in the head and neck region, including the oral cavity and oropharynx.[16] Oral cancer and oropharyngeal cancer are two distinctive entities clinically, histopathologically, and genetically.[17] This article focuses on oral cancer. The most common sites of oral SCC (OSCC) are the tongue and floor of mouth, which account for more than 50% of all the cases, followed by the gingiva, palatal mucosa, and buccal and labial mucosa.[18] OSCC usually progresses rapidly, and the prognosis is closely associated with the tumor staging.[19] In the United States, approximately 50% of the OSCC patients present with regional or distant metastasis at the time of diagnosis.[20] OSCC tumors can double in size within three months, which clinically equates to a T1 tumor progressing to a T3 tumor in less than two years.[21] This accelerated progression corresponds to a dismal prognosis. The overall 5-year survival rate of OSCC is approximately 60%, varying between 80% for stage I cancers and 40% for stage IV cancers.[3]

Treatment strategies for OSCC vary based on the stage at time of diagnosis. Patients with localized disease typically receive surgery and/or radiotherapy, leading to a high probability of long-term survival but with considerable morbidity.[22] With metastatic OSCC, chemotherapy and radiotherapy are the mainstays of treatment.[22] Recently, targeted therapeutics have been introduced into treatment regimens or ongoing clinical trials to improve survival rate and reduce toxicity, such as cetuximab (monoclonal epidermal growth factor receptor [EGFR] antibody), bevacizumab (monoclonal vascular endothelial growth factor [VEGF] antibody), and mechanistic target of rapamycin (mTOR) inhibitors.[22] With the advancement of immunotherapy, monoclonal antibodies that target programmed cell death protein-1 (PD-1), a receptor of the immune escape pathway, such as nivolumab and pembrolizumab, have been approved by the Food and Drug Administration (FDA) for recurrent and/or metastatic head and neck SCC.[22]

Despite the progress in investigating the pathobiological mechanisms of OSCC, the prognosis has unfortunately not improved over the past few decades.[23] This is largely due to the frequent occurrence of local and regional OSCC recurrences as well as high morbidity and mortality rates.[23] The clinical challenge remains in accurately detecting regional metastasis and efficiently treating second primary OSCC and recurrent tumors.[23] This article reviews our understanding of the etiopathologic mechanisms of OSCC from both genetic and epigenetic perspectives and discusses the role of precision medicine in OSCC prevention, detection, and management.

INITIATION AND PROGRESSION OF ORAL SQUAMOUS CELL CARCINOMA
Initiation of Oral Squamous Cell Carcinoma—Field Cancerization

Most OSCC tumors develop from an existing premalignant lesion, such as leukoplakia, erythroplakia, or proliferative verrucous leukoplakia.[24] In addition, OSCC is notorious for its high recurrence rate and the frequent occurrence of synchronous and/or metachronous primary tumors.[23] To explain this clinical phenomenon and aid our understanding of OSCC initiation, Slaughter and colleagues[25] proposed the concept of "field cancerization." Field cancerization refers to the formation of large, preneoplastic fields of carcinogen-exposed mucosal epithelium that are not apparent on clinical or histologic examination. The process of field cancerization occurs at the molecular level. Cells acquire and accumulate a series of genetic or epigenetic alterations that lead to cell cycle dysregulation and uncontrolled cell proliferation, ultimately predisposing these cells toward malignant transformation.[24]

Field cancerization is a multistep process and has been described in many organ systems, such as oral epithelium, esophagus, and skin.[26,27] The precancerized fields in OSCC have been characterized based on the expression of a mutated tumor suppressor, p53.[27] This is caused by loss-of-function mutations of the gene *TP53* that encodes the tumor protein p53.[27] Initially, cells with *TP53* loss-of-function mutation form a patch, suggesting its clonal nature. These patches gradually expand by acquiring additional mutations, allowing for advantages toward cell proliferation, and eventually form a confluent preneoplastic field that displaces the normal epithelium.[28]

Initiation of Oral Squamous Cell Carcinoma—Cancer-initiating Cells in Oral Squamous Cell Carcinoma

Similar to other solid tumors, OSCC exhibits tumor heterogeneity.[29] OSCC is thought to begin with a specialized population of cancer-initiating cells (CICs)/cancer stem cells (CSCs), which possess stemness, or the ability to self-renew and generate heterogeneous clones of neoplastic cells that form a precancerized field and ultimately comprise the tumor.[30,31] Multiple hypotheses have been proposed to explain the origin of CICs, such as epigenetically altered normal tissue stem cells or dedifferentiated tumor cells.[32] More research needs to be done to clarify the origin of CICs in OSCC. CICs are slow-cycling cells and are resistant to conventional chemotherapeutics that target highly proliferative cells.[33] Thus, CICs are able to avoid cell death after chemotherapy and utilize their stem cell–like features to regenerate the whole tumor mass and cause a recurrence.[24,30]

Putative CICs of OSCCs have been defined by cell surface markers (eg, CD133 and CD44) or based on Hoechst dye exclusion (eg, side population), followed by xenograft transplantation assays.[33–36] These experiments, however, only demonstrated the ability of a defined population of OSCC cells to form tumors in a new environment and did not necessarily recapitulate the behavior of such cancer cells in their native environment. Thus, these studies provided little molecular insight into the mechanism by which CICs self-renew or differentiate into different cancer clones. Studies suggest that CICs can be more accurately defined and studied in intact tumors by lineage tracing and clonal analysis.[37–39] This in vivo approach typically involves a Cre recombinase-based cell type-specific fluorescent labeling. Cancer cells can be permanently labeled and tracked based on known stem cell markers (eg, Lgr5 promoter for intestinal crypt stem cells).[40] B-cell specific Moloney murine leukemia virus insertion site 1 (Bmi1), a transcription repressor, plays a critical role in cell senescence.[41] By applying the lineage tracing strategy, Bmi1+ cells can be visualized in the basal cell layer of normal lingual epithelium, regulating tissue maintenance and regeneration.[42] Recent studies revealed that Bmi1+ subpopulation in OSCC was a subset of slow-cycling tumor propagating cells and mediated invasive growth and regional metastasis of OSCC.[43,44] Eliminating Bmi1+ OSCC cells significantly reduced the occurrence of metastasis, indicating the potential therapeutic value of Bmi1 inhibitors in OSCC treatments.[44]

Multistep Progression of Oral Squamous Cell Carcinoma

The multistep progression of OSCC involves an accumulation of both genetic and epigenetic alterations in oncogenes or tumor suppressor genes, leading to cell cycle dysregulation, inhibition of growth suppressors, and resistance to apoptosis (**Fig. 1**).[45,46] Meanwhile, the interactions between tumor cells and microenvironment enhance the progression and invasion of OSCC.

The role of chromosomal instability (eg, telomerase dysfunction and loss of heterozygosity [LOH]) in the process of malignant transformation has been studied extensively.[46] Telomeres are G-rich proteins at the distal ends of chromosomes that play a critical role in maintaining cell cycle homeostasis.[47] Telomerase is a telomere-specific polymerase that maintains telomere integrity by its functional subunit, telomerase reverse transcriptase (TERT), to synthesize the telomere sequences.[47] Mutations of TERT, which have been detected in 80% of OSCC tumors, lead to cell cycle dysregulation and uncontrolled cell proliferation.[48] It is unclear, however, if there is an association between TERT mutations and patient outcome. In addition to telomerase dysfunction, LOH of chromosomes 3p, 8p, 9p (p16), and 17p (p53) are often key events in OSCC initiation and progression.[48] LOH refers to the loss of chromosomal regions containing a gene (eg, tumor suppressor gene) in either the maternal or paternal allele, resulting in higher tumor susceptibility.[48] Specifically, LOH at 17p13 (p53 locus) is significantly associated with the higher incidence of OSCC development.[49] *TP53* gene, known as the "guardian of the genome," plays an essential role in cell cycle regulation and DNA damage-induced apoptosis (**Fig. 2**).[48,50] Up to 80% of OSCC tumors exhibit *TP53* inactivation, typically through point mutations, which are single-nucleotide mutations in the DNA sequence.[51,52] Inactivation of p53 can further cause cell immortalization.[53] Mutations of *CDKN2A*, *CCND1*, *PIK3CA*, *PTEN*, and *HRAS* can also cause cell cycle dysregulation and immortalization, and are associated with OSCC initiation and progression (see **Fig. 2**).[50–52] The tumor suppressor gene, *CDKN2A*, encodes the p16 protein that regulates cell cycle progression.[54] Deletion or inactivation of *CDKN2A* is associated with cell immortalization and is seen in approximately 50% of OSCC tumors.[54] Cyclin D1, a protein encoded by the *CCND1* gene, allows for progression through the cell cycle.[53] *CCND1* amplification leads to cell proliferation and is identified in 20% to 30% of OSCCs.[52,54] Upon binding with its ligand, EGFR, a transmembrane receptor tyrosine kinase, functions to regulate cell proliferation, survival, and apoptosis via multiple downstream signaling pathways (eg, PI3K/AKT pathway and Ras/Raf/mitogen-activated protein kinase [MAPK] pathway).[55,56] PIK3CA, a catalytic subunit of phosphatidylinositol 3-kinases (PI3K), is recruited by EGFR to activate the downstream survival cascade. The activity of PI3K is regulated by the tumor suppressor, phosphatase and tensin homolog (PTEN).[56] Inactivated or deleted PTEN enhances cell survival, migration, and angiogenesis via PIK3CA and AKT activation.[48] Amplification of PIK3CA and EGFR is present in 27% and 14% of OSCC tumors, respectively.[54,57] In addition, *NOTCH1*

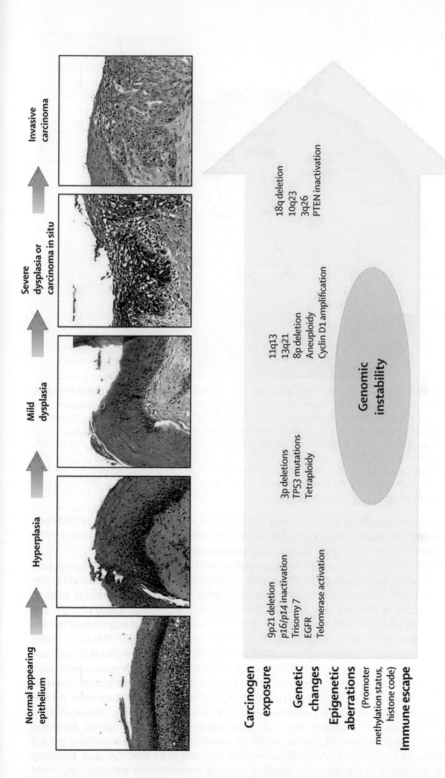

Fig. 1. Oral carcinogenesis is a complex multistep process characterized by an accumulation of genetic and epigenetic alterations, leading to genomic instability.[45] Histopathologic progression of OSCC is presented in hematoxylin-eosin stain (×200).[45] (*From* Agriris A, Karamouzis MV, Raben D, et al. Head and neck cancer. Lancet 2008;371[9625]:1696; with permission.)

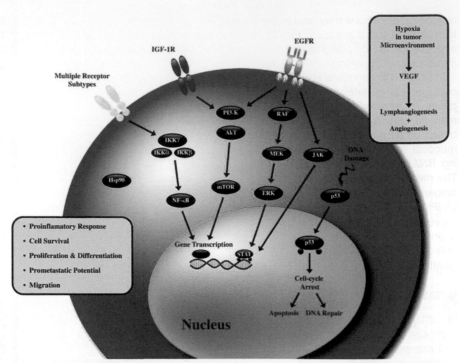

Fig. 2. Altered regulatory signaling pathways (eg, PI3K/AKT pathway and Ras/Raf/MAPK pathway) and inactivated p53 cause cell-cycle dysregulation and cell immortalization and contribute to the initiation and progression of OSCC.[50] ERK, extracellular signal–related kinase; Hsp90, heat shock protein 90; IGF-1R, insulinlike growth factor-1 receptor; IKKα, inhibitor κB kinase alpha; IKKβ, inhibitor κB kinase beta; IKKγ, inhibitor κB kinase gamma; JAK, Janus kinase; MEK, MAPK/ERK kinase; NF, nuclear factor; STAT, signal transducers and activators of transcription.[50] (*From* Stadler ME, Patel MR, Couch ME, et al. Molecular biology of head and neck cancer: risks and pathways. Hematol Oncol Clin North Am 2008;22:1106, vii; with permission.)

loss-of-function mutations are detected in 15% of OSCC tumors.[51,52,54] NOTCH1 regulates skin differentiation and homeostasis, and conditional *NOTCH1* knockout mice develop skin tumors, indicating its role as a tumor suppressor protein.[58]

Epigenetic alterations, such as DNA methylation and histone modifications, regulate gene expression by adjusting chromosomal structures as opposed to changing the DNA sequence.[59] Aberrant promoter hypermethylation interrupts the binding of transcription factors to the promoter of key tumor suppressor genes, leading to silencing of these genes and promotion of tumor growth.[60,61] Transcriptional silencing of the tumor suppressor gene, p16, is detected in 50% to 75% of OSCC tumors.[62–64] Many epigenetic drugs have been developed to effectively reverse DNA methylation that occurs in cancer. DNA methylation inhibitors were the first epigenetic drugs proposed for use as cancer therapeutics.[65] Research has also shown global DNA hypomethylation in OSCC tumors despite the regional promoter hypermethylation.[66] Moreover, the degree of global hypomethylation is enhanced in the advanced stage of OSCC.[66] Histones are structural proteins that are packaged with DNA into a complex organization. Histone modifications, such as acetylation and methylation, induce conformational changes of DNA molecules and regulate the transcriptional activities by either exposing or blocking the binding sites of transcription factors.[67] Aberrant histone modifications may lead to the abnormal transcriptional activity and contribute to malignant transformation (**Fig. 3**).[67,68] For example, recent studies revealed that hypoacetylation of H3K9ac is associated with cell proliferation and epithelial-to-mesenchymal transition (EMT) in OSCC.[69]

In addition to genetic and epigenetic alterations, microRNAs (miRNAs) contribute to oncogenesis by altering the expression of tumor suppressor genes and/or onco-genes.[70] The significance of miRNAs as a group of robust prognostic indicators in human cancers has long been recognized.[71] Molecular characterization of OSCCs based on 61 miRNAs achieved 93% accuracy to distinguish normal and malignant mucosal epithelium.[72] miRNAs are 18–23 nucleotide-long, single-stranded, noncoding RNAs that function as post-transcriptional repressors of their target genes.[73] The mechanisms that alter miRNA expression include transcriptional dysregulation, epigenetic modifications, chromosomal changes, single nucleotide polymorphisms (SNPs), and defects in the processing machinery.[74,75] An miRNA may regulate the expression of multiple targeted mRNA molecules.[76] Many altered miRNAs have been linked with the pathogenesis of OSCC.[70] For example, down-regulation of miR-375 is commonly seen in OSCC, and functional restoration of miR-375 can significantly suppress tumor aggressiveness, suggesting its role as a tumor suppressor.[70]

METASTASIS OF ORAL SQUAMOUS CELL CARCINOMA

Metastasis of cancer cells is one of the major prognostic indicators in OSCC.[46] Typically, metastatic tumors of OSCC present in the cervical lymph nodes and are associated with poor clinical prognosis.[46,77] The model of EMT provides

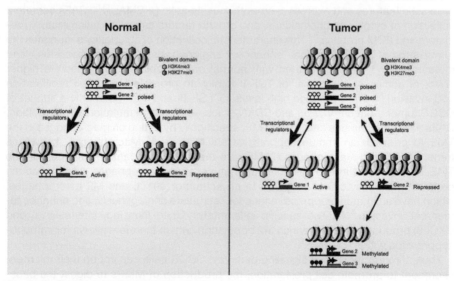

Fig. 3. (*Left*) In normal stem cells, many genes remain bivalent marks (ie, both active [H3K4me3] and repressed [H3K27me3]) at the promoter regions on the chromosomes. During normal development, this poised state will transform into either an active or repressed state to regulate gene expression. (*Right*) In cancer cells, the determined state can be reversed to bivalent state, and cells regain cellular plasticity (ie, dedifferentiation). In certain differentiation-related genes, the promoters are hypermethylated, leading to a permanently silenced state.[68] (*From* Easwaran H, Tsai HC, Baylin SB. Cancer epigenetics: tumor heterogeneity, plasticity of stem-like states, and drug resistance. Mol Cell 2014;54:720; with permission.)

an appealing hypothesis to explain this extremely complex multistep process.[78] EMT refers to the transdifferentiation program of epithelial cells into motile mesenchymal cells that allow for growth and invasion. With the loss of cell polarity and cell-cell adhesion molecules (eg, E-cadherin), OSCC cells acquire mesenchymal features, such as motile phenotypes and expression of mesenchymal markers (eg, N-cadherin and vimentin).[78] In addition, there are constant interactions between OSCC cells and the surrounding microenvironment that also promote metastasis.[79]

Although the molecular mechanism of EMT is not yet fully understood, it is known to rely on paracrine signaling between the tumor cells and the surrounding tumor microenvironment (TME).[80] The TME is composed of stromal cells, immune cells, and the surrounding extracellular matrix (ECM).[80] One of the most prominent and extensively studied signaling pathways associated with EMT is the transforming growth factor β (TGF-β) pathway. TGF-β functions by binding to TGF-β receptors I and II, which are serine/threonine kinases that mediate intracellular signaling pathways via SMAD proteins.[81] The complex then can translocate into the nucleus to alter gene expression.[81] TGF-βI and TGF-βII also stimulate the synthesis of Snail (SNAI1) and Slug (SNAI2), two transcription factors that have been shown to drive EMT by leading to the loss of E-cadherin expression.[82] TGF-β is also known to promote tumor invasion by increasing the expression of matrix metalloproteinases (MMPs), including MMP-1, MMP-3, MMP-9, and MMP-10.[81] In addition, TGF-β has been shown to promote the transition of stromal cells into cancer-associated fibroblasts (CAFs), which also play a prominent role in EMT and metastasis.[83]

Fibroblasts in the TME are capable of transforming into CAFs, which exhibit myofibroblastic features and express α–smooth muscle actin (α-SMA).[83,84] CAFs secrete a collection of cytokines, chemokines, and growth factors as well as inflammatory mediators and ECM proteins.[83] This characteristic collection of chemokines mediates the tumor-stromal cross-talk that enhances angiogenesis, lymphangiogenesis, and metastasis.[84,85] When compared with normal oral fibroblasts, CAFs secrete higher levels of activin A, a member of TGF-β family, to promote tumor cell proliferation and invasion.[83] CAFs produce high levels of TGF-βI and TGF-βII in only a subset of OSCC tumors that carry TP53 and CDKN2A loss-of-function mutations.[86] In addition, CAFs affect the immune cells in the TME, specifically by acting on macrophages in the TME to promote an immunosuppressive environment.[87] Macrophages, known as tumor-associated macrophages (TAMs), are the most abundant immune cells in the TME.[87] TAMs exist in two functional phenotypes: M1 macrophages, which produce proinflammatory cytokines that lead to an antitumor effect; and M2 macrophages, which have an immunosuppressive function, stimulate angiogenesis, and enhance tumor cell invasion.[87,88] The specific inflammatory cytokines (eg, interleukin-6 and CXCL8) produced by CAFs enrich M2 population, which therefore allows for immunosuppression within the TME.[87]

Thus, through the TGF-β signaling pathway, OSCC cells can act on their microenvironment to promote cell proliferation, the production of MMPs to digest the basement membrane, and the transformation of oral fibroblasts into CAFs. These interactions further promote metastasis, local immunosuppression, and tumor invasion.

OMICS TECHNOLOGY IN UNDERSTANDING THE PATHOBIOLOGICAL MECHANISMS OF ORAL SQUAMOUS CELL CARCINOMA

To obtain the most optimal patient outcome, medical care strategies in cancer medicine include effective prevention, early detection, and diagnosis as well as efficacious treatment with minimal toxicities. In this post-genomics era, our understanding of cancer pathobiology has gradually transitioned from a morphology-based to a genetics-based system.[89] As discussed previously, OSCC is a complex genetic disease exhibiting tumor heterogeneity and tumor plasticity.[29] Medical care decisions need to be customized based on the unique genomic and proteomic features of each individual tumor. To address OSCC tumor heterogeneity and individual variations, current research uses omics technologies, such as genomics, transcriptomics, proteomics, and metabolomics, with the goal of identifying biomarkers based on tumor biopsies, circulating tumor cells, or body fluid (eg, saliva).[90] Omics technologies are high-throughput screening methodologies that can qualitatively and quantitatively analyze target molecules (eg, transcripts) in one experiment.[91] Unlike conventional cancer genetic research that addresses one or a few signaling pathways at a time, omics technologies provide a comprehensive and unbiased overview of the genome-scale or proteome-scale data sets.[91] With the aid of bioinformatics, an enormous amount of information is generated, and the complex, clinically meaningful effects can, therefore, be uncovered. The integration of omics technologies, bioinformatics, and conventional molecular biology has dramatically changed the landscape of cancer research and has a great impact on the understanding of the disease process.[92] Furthermore, with its improved accuracy and efficiency, omics technologies now have extended their role to molecular diagnostics and biomarker discovery.[91] The recent applications of omics technologies in investigating the pathobiological mechanisms of OSCC are reviewed.

Genomics in Oral Squamous Cell Carcinoma Research

Genomics-related technology includes whole-genome sequencing and whole-exome sequencing. There are multiple commercial platforms available for identifying gene mutations, SNPs, or copy number alterations.[91] The Cancer Genome Atlas (TCGA), launched in 2005, is a collaboration between the National Cancer Institute (NCI) and the National Human Genome Research Institute.[93] TCGA has generated comprehensive, multidimensional maps of key genomic changes in thirty-three types of cancer, including head and neck SCC.[93] The comprehensive genomic profiling has revealed two distinct subtypes of oral and oropharyngeal SCC: HPV-negative tumors, which typically arise in oral cavity proper and lips; and HPV-positive tumors, which mainly present in the oropharynx.[51,52,93] These two subtypes of SCC harbor distinct molecular alterations that correspond to their clinical behavior and patient prognosis.[93] Consistent with prior studies, the TCGA database revealed that a vast majority of HPV-negative OSCCs exhibit *TP53* loss-of-function mutations and *CDKN2A* inactivation.[93] In addition, integrated genomic analyses indicated a high level of heterogeneity in HPV-negative OSCC.[93] Novel mutations overlooked in the previous studies were discovered using whole-exome sequencing, a transcriptomics technique for sequencing all of the expressed genes in a genome (known as the exome).[51,52] Mutations in *NOTCH1* occurred in approximately 15% of cases, and mutations and focal copy-number alterations of *NOTCH2/3* were detected in the additional 11% of OSCC cases.[51,52]

The astonishing heterogeneity of OSCC illustrates how precision medicine can truly benefit patients and improve medical care. Further advancing from whole-exome sequencing to whole-genome sequencing, the PanCancer Analysis of Whole Genomes project (PCAWG) is now steered to reveal noncoding driver mutations, including alternative promoter usage, splicing, expression, editing, fusion, allele-specific expression, and nonsynonymous variants.[94] These noncoding transcripts, namely miRNAs and long noncoding RNAs (lncRNAs), demonstrate a tremendous potential for further clinical inquiries.[95,96]

Transcriptomics in Oral Squamous Cell Carcinoma Research

Extensive efforts have been distributed to characterize OSCC at the molecular level with transcriptomics technology.[97] To improve the therapeutic regimens for the managements of OSCC, reliable biomarkers are required to facilitate the prediction of clinical outcome and monitor treatment efficacy. When surveying a cohort of OSCC transcriptomes, dysregulation of multiple pathways (eg, mRNA processing, cytoskeletal organization, metabolic processes, cell cycle regulation, and apoptosis) was detected.[97] Similar to lung SCC, molecular characterization of OSCC has also been proposed.[98] Affected signaling pathways include dysregulation of the KEAP1/NFE2L2 oxidative stress pathway, differential utilization of the lineage markers SOX2 and TP63, and PIK3CA and EGFR mutations.[98] Clinically distinct behaviors are associated with different activation patterns of the EGFR pathway.[99] A molecular signature has also been proposed to predict the presence of lymph node metastases using the primary tumor at the time of diagnosis to assist in treatment planning for OSCC.[99,100] In addition, microarray data revealed the overexpression of BGH3, MMP9, and PDIA3 in more than 80% of OSCC tumors, suggesting the importance of ECM-cell receptor interactions in OSCC progression.[101] For potential clinical applications, these transcriptional signatures can be complementary in facilitating the formation of personalized therapeutic regimens in the management of OSCC.

Proteomics and Phospho-proteomics in Oral Squamous Cell Carcinoma Research

A landmark study in 2011 measuring the absolute mRNA and protein abundance and turnover by parallel metabolic pulse labeling revealed that cellular abundance of proteins is predominantly controlled by the level of translation.[102] Although mRNA and protein levels do correlate to a certain extent, genome-wide protein abundance is still a crucial parameter to understand cellular state and function. High-throughput analyses of both total and phosphorylated proteins allow for investigation of intracellular and secreted proteins in body fluid specimens (eg, serum, plasma, urine, and saliva).[103] Proteomic analysis, complemented with in situ hybridization or immunohistochemistry, has revealed altered expression at the protein level in cell metabolism, adhesion, motility, and signal transduction.[104–106] Studies have demonstrated promising results in distinguishing OSCC and normal samples by salivary or serum proteomics analyses with sensitivity and specificity as high as 80% to 90%.[106,107]

Metabolomics and Lipidomics in Oral Squamous Cell Carcinoma Research

Aided by mass spectrometry-based metabolomics analysis, metabolite profiling of tissue and body fluid specimens with the goal of biomarker discovery in OSCC research has revealed significant changes in energy metabolism pathways (eg, glycolysis and tricarboxylic acid cycle).[108] In the serum specimens from OSCC patients, the level of glycolytic metabolites (eg, glucose) are higher, with lower levels of certain amino acids (ie, valine, tyrosine, serine, and methionine).[109] On the contrary, such metabolite expression patterns are reversed in OSCC tumor tissues, suggesting the clinical implication of this signature panel as a screening tool.[109] Furthermore, OSCC cells can be subclassified into different groups based on their metabolic phenotypes (pyruvate, succinic acid, malic acid, citric acid, fumaric acid, and alphaketoglutaric acid) using high performance ion chromatography.[110] The clinical correlations discovered in these early studies, however, need to be validated by well-designed experiments. Lipids have also been identified as an important class of metabolites, and altered circulatory cholesterol levels have been linked to multiple cancer types.[111–113] It was reported that the levels of total lipids, cholesterol, and high-density lipoprotein were significantly lower in OSCC patients compared with healthy controls.[113,114] Although still primitive, these lipidomic data may suggest increased utilization by neoplastic cells for new membrane biogenesis and warrant further investigation.

With the rapid development of the omics tools discussed previously, these technologies will be collectively powerful with the potential to reveal molecular mechanisms and crucial signaling pathways driving the disease. In addition, these tools can be used to pinpoint novel therapeutic targets as well as nominate biomarkers that can be utilized in cancer diagnosis, prognosis prediction, and treatment surveillance.

FROM SCIENCE TO MEDICINE: THE INTEGRATION AND APPLICATION OF BIG DATA ON PERSONALIZED MANAGEMENTS OF ORAL CANCER

Based on the definition provided by the NCI, precision medicine, also known as personalized medicine, is "an approach to patient care that allows doctors to select treatments that are most likely to help patients based on a genetic understanding of their disease."[115] With the evolution of omics technologies, a large amount of information has been gained from the molecular profiling of OSCC tumors. Clinicians and scientists are expected to collaborate and translate these findings into medication targets for treating OSCC.[116] Typically, cancer-specific cell receptors or intracellular signaling molecules are targeted by either monoclonal antibodies (eg, cetuximab) or synthetic small molecules (eg, gefinitib).[22] Omics data addressing molecular changes alone, however, are insufficient to implement genomics-based precision medicine.[92] More importantly, we need to understand how these aberrant genes contribute to the tumor behaviors (eg, determinant of metastasis, response to a particular drug). It is known that omics data harbor a noisy mixture of cancer-causing mutations and bystander mutations.[117] Thus, in addition to generating cancer genomic data, more efforts should be directed to the identification and functional validation of the cancer-causing mutations.

After candidate mutation discovery by omics-scale methods, the next crucial step is to generate a clinically relevant hypothesis and design well-controlled experiments in tissue culture or animal models to validate the role of each candidate mutation in the cancer-related activities, such as invasiveness and interactions with the surrounding microenvironment.[118,119] In addition, it is critical to correlate experimental data with clinical presentations and confirm the expression of target mutations in human specimens by immunohistochemistry, fluorescence in situ hybridization (FISH), or gene expression microarray.[115] In the beginning of the biomarker discovery and drug design process, it is also important to characterize the biochemical and structural features of the target protein. Thus, we can screen based on the activity of compounds in a library, and then optimize its drug-like property and measure its potency, specificity, and pharmacokinetic characteristics. Initiatives by national and international consortia, such as the Cancer Therapy Evaluation Program organized by the NCI and International Cancer Genomics Consortium, coordinate resources and efforts to investigate comprehensive molecular profiling for multiple cancer types, as well as develop and assess novel targeted anticancer drugs and sponsor clinical trials.[120] Thus far, there are four large-scale head and neck cancer projects globally and in the United States.[120] Finally, ethical considerations derived from the medical advancement (eg, privacy, confidentiality, and potential possibility for discrimination) also need to be addressed.[120] Readers are referred to the published guidelines and recommendations for detailed regulations.[121]

SUMMARY

OSCC is a distinct subtype of head and neck SCC with traditional risk factors, such as tobacco, alcohol, and areca nut. These cancers are predominantly HPV negative and harbor *TP53* loss-of-function mutations. Although there are now highly sophisticated diagnostic systems, OSCCs are primarily treated with surgical excision and cervical lymph node dissection, both of which are associated with high morbidity and mortality. Prognosis remains dismal with an approximately 50% 5-year survival rate for advanced OSCC tumors. OSCCs are heterogeneous tumors with genetic and epigenetic aberrations, encompassing a wide range of oncogenic pathways (eg, PI3K-PTEN-AKT-mTOR). With the advent of genomic, proteomic, and metabolomic profiling, comprehensive biomarkers have been discovered that can identify tumors with greater invasive and metastatic potential. Investigation of new and currently identified biomarkers in the validation cohorts and multicenter clinical trials will further pave the way for developing truly personalized therapy for OSCC patients.

REFERENCES

1. Ferlay J, Soerjomataram I, Dikshit R, et al. Cancer incidence and mortality worldwide: sources, methods and major patterns in GLOBOCAN 2012. Int J Cancer 2015;136:E359–86.
2. Warnakulasuriya S. Living with oral cancer: epidemiology with particular reference to prevalence and life-style changes that influence survival. Oral Oncol 2010;46:407–10.
3. Siegel RL, Miller KD, Jemal A. Cancer statistics, 2016. CA Cancer J Clin 2016; 66:7–30.
4. Siegel R, Ma J, Zou Z, et al. Cancer statistics, 2014. CA Cancer J Clin 2014; 64(1):9–29.
5. Siegel R, Naishadham D, Jemal A. Cancer statistics, 2013. CA Cancer J Clin 2013;63:11–30.
6. Siegel R, Naishadham D, Jemal A. Cancer statistics, 2012. CA Cancer J Clin 2012;62:10–29.
7. Siegel R, Ward E, Brawley O, et al. Cancer statistics, 2011: the impact of eliminating socioeconomic and racial disparities on premature cancer deaths. CA Cancer J Clin 2011;61:212–36.
8. Jemal A, Siegel R, Xu J, et al. Cancer statistics, 2010. CA Cancer J Clin 2010;60: 277–300.
9. de Camargo Cancela M, de Souza DL, Curado MP. International incidence of oropharyngeal cancer: a population-based study. Oral Oncol 2012;48:484–90.
10. D'Souza G, Kreimer AR, Viscidi R, et al. Case-control study of human papillomavirus and oropharyngeal cancer. N Engl J Med 2007;356:1944–56.
11. Ang KK, Harris J, Wheeler R, et al. Human papillomavirus and survival of patients with oropharyngeal cancer. N Engl J Med 2010;363:24–35.
12. McBride KA, Ballinger ML, Killick E, et al. Li-Fraumeni syndrome: cancer risk assessment and clinical management. Nat Rev Clin Oncol 2014;11:260–71.
13. Romick-Rosendale LE, Lui VW, Grandis JR, et al. The Fanconi anemia pathway: repairing the link between DNA damage and squamous cell carcinoma. Mutat Res 2013;743-744:78–88.

14. Kutler DI, Auerbach AD, Satagopan J, et al. High incidence of head and neck squamous cell carcinoma in patients with Fanconi anemia. Arch Otolaryngol Head Neck Surg 2003;129:106–12.

15. Scully C, Langdon J, Evans J. Marathon of eponyms: 26 Zinsser-Engman-Cole syndrome (Dyskeratosis congenita). Oral Dis 2012;18:522–3.

16. Chen YK, Huang HC, Lin LM, et al. Primary oral squamous cell carcinoma: an analysis of 703 cases in southern Taiwan. Oral Oncol 1999;35:173–9.

17. Seiwert TY, Zuo Z, Keck MK, et al. Integrative and comparative genomic analysis of HPV-positive and HPV-negative head and neck squamous cell carcinomas. Clin Cancer Res 2015;21:632–41.

18. Bagan J, Sarrion G, Jimenez Y. Oral cancer: clinical features. Oral Oncol 2010; 46:414–7.

19. Warnakulasuriya S. Global epidemiology of oral and oropharyngeal cancer. Oral Oncol 2009;45:309–16.

20. Massano J, Regateiro FS, Januario G, et al. Oral squamous cell carcinoma: review of prognostic and predictive factors. Oral Surg Oral Med Oral Pathol Oral Radiol Endod 2006;102:67–76.

21. Goy J, Hall SF, Feldman-Stewart D, et al. Diagnostic delay and disease stage in head and neck cancer: a systematic review. Laryngoscope 2009;119:889–98.

22. Algazi AP, Grandis JR. Head and neck cancer in 2016: a watershed year for improvements in treatment? Nat Rev Clin Oncol 2017;14:76–8.

23. Schmitz S, Ang KK, Vermorken J, et al. Targeted therapies for squamous cell carcinoma of the head and neck: current knowledge and future directions. Cancer Treat Rev 2014;40:390–404.

24. Feller LL, Khammissa RR, Kramer BB, et al. Oral squamous cell carcinoma in relation to field precancerisation: pathobiology. Cancer Cell Int 2013;13:31.

25. Slaughter DP, Southwick HW, Smejkal W. Field cancerization in oral stratified squamous epithelium; clinical implications of multicentric origin. Cancer 1953; 6:963–8.

26. Simple M, Suresh A, Das D, et al. Cancer stem cells and field cancerization of oral squamous cell carcinoma. Oral Oncol 2015;51:643–51.

27. Braakhuis BJ, Tabor MP, Kummer JA, et al. A genetic explanation of Slaughter's concept of field cancerization: evidence and clinical implications. Cancer Res 2003;63:1727–30.

28. van Houten VM, Tabor MP, van den Brekel MW, et al. Mutated p53 as a molecular marker for the diagnosis of head and neck cancer. J Pathol 2002;198: 476–86.

29. Stucky A, Sedghizadeh PP, Mahabady S, et al. Single-cell genomic analysis of head and neck squamous cell carcinoma. Oncotarget 2017.

30. Sayed SI, Dwivedi RC, Katna R, et al. Implications of understanding cancer stem cell (CSC) biology in head and neck squamous cell cancer. Oral Oncol 2011;47:237–43.

31. Ehrensberger AH, Svejstrup JQ. Reprogramming chromatin. Crit Rev Biochem Mol Biol 2012;47:464–82.

32. Bjerkvig R, Tysnes BB, Aboody KS, et al. Opinion: the origin of the cancer stem cell: current controversies and new insights. Nat Rev Cancer 2005;5:899–904.

33. Prince ME, Sivanandan R, Kaczorowski A, et al. Identification of a subpopulation of cells with cancer stem cell properties in head and neck squamous cell carcinoma. Proc Natl Acad Sci U S A 2007;104:973–8.

34. Chen YS, Wu MJ, Huang CY, et al. CD133/Src axis mediates tumor initiating property and epithelial-mesenchymal transition of head and neck cancer. PLoS One 2011;6:e28053.
35. Clay MR, Tabor M, Owen JH, et al. Single-marker identification of head and neck squamous cell carcinoma cancer stem cells with aldehyde dehydrogenase. Head Neck 2010;32:1195–201.
36. Joshua B, Kaplan MJ, Doweck I, et al. Frequency of cells expressing CD44, a head and neck cancer stem cell marker: correlation with tumor aggressiveness. Head Neck 2012;34:42–9.
37. Weissman TA, Pan YA. Brainbow: new resources and emerging biological applications for multicolor genetic labeling and analysis. Genetics 2015;199: 293–306.
38. Driessens G, Beck B, Caauwe A, et al. Defining the mode of tumour growth by clonal analysis. Nature 2012;488:527–30.
39. Singh AK, Arya RK, Maheshwari S, et al. Tumor heterogeneity and cancer stem cell paradigm: updates in concept, controversies and clinical relevance. Int J Cancer 2015;136:1991–2000.
40. Schepers AG, Snippert HJ, Stange DE, et al. Lineage tracing reveals Lgr5+ stem cell activity in mouse intestinal adenomas. Science 2012;337:730–5.
41. Park IK, Morrison SJ, Clarke MF. Bmi1, stem cells, and senescence regulation. J Clin Invest 2004;113:175–9.
42. Tanaka T, Komai Y, Tokuyama Y, et al. Identification of stem cells that maintain and regenerate lingual keratinized epithelial cells. Nat Cell Biol 2013;15:511–8.
43. Tanaka T, Atsumi N, Nakamura N, et al. Bmi1-positive cells in the lingual epithelium could serve as cancer stem cells in tongue cancer. Sci Rep 2016;6:39386.
44. Chen D, Wu M, Li Y, et al. Targeting BMI1+ cancer stem cells overcomes chemoresistance and inhibits metastases in squamous cell carcinoma. Cell Stem Cell 2017;20:621–34.e6.
45. Argiris A, Karamouzis MV, Raben D, et al. Head and neck cancer. Lancet 2008; 371:1695–709.
46. Haddad RI, Shin DM. Recent advances in head and neck cancer. N Engl J Med 2008;359:1143–54.
47. Benhamou Y, Picco V, Pages G. The telomere proteins in tumorigenesis and clinical outcomes of oral squamous cell carcinoma. Oral Oncol 2016;57:46–53.
48. Leemans CR, Braakhuis BJ, Brakenhoff RH. The molecular biology of head and neck cancer. Nat Rev Cancer 2011;11:9–22.
49. Partridge M, Pateromichelakis S, Phillips E, et al. A case-control study confirms that microsatellite assay can identify patients at risk of developing oral squamous cell carcinoma within a field of cancerization. Cancer Res 2000;60: 3893–8.
50. Stadler ME, Patel MR, Couch ME, et al. Molecular biology of head and neck cancer: risks and pathways. Hematol Oncol Clin North Am 2008;22:1099–124, vii.
51. Agrawal N, Frederick MJ, Pickering CR, et al. Exome sequencing of head and neck squamous cell carcinoma reveals inactivating mutations in NOTCH1. Science 2011;333:1154–7.
52. Stransky N, Egloff AM, Tward AD, et al. The mutational landscape of head and neck squamous cell carcinoma. Science 2011;333:1157–60.
53. Opitz OG, Suliman Y, Hahn WC, et al. Cyclin D1 overexpression and p53 inactivation immortalize primary oral keratinocytes by a telomerase-independent mechanism. J Clin Invest 2001;108:725–32.

54. Chung CH, Guthrie VB, Masica DL, et al. Genomic alterations in head and neck squamous cell carcinoma determined by cancer gene-targeted sequencing. Ann Oncol 2015;26:1216–23.

55. Ongkeko WM, Altuna X, Weisman RA, et al. Expression of protein tyrosine kinases in head and neck squamous cell carcinomas. Am J Clin Pathol 2005; 124:71–6.

56. Choi S, Myers JN. Molecular pathogenesis of oral squamous cell carcinoma: implications for therapy. J Dent Res 2008;87:14–32.

57. Murugan AK, Hong NT, Fukui Y, et al. Oncogenic mutations of the PIK3CA gene in head and neck squamous cell carcinomas. Int J Oncol 2008;32:101–11.

58. Nicolas M, Wolfer A, Raj K, et al. Notch1 functions as a tumor suppressor in mouse skin. Nat Genet 2003;33:416–21.

59. Egger G, Liang G, Aparicio A, et al. Epigenetics in human disease and prospects for epigenetic therapy. Nature 2004;429:457–63.

60. Gasche JA, Goel A. Epigenetic mechanisms in oral carcinogenesis. Future Oncol 2012;8:1407–25.

61. Jithesh PV, Risk JM, Schache AG, et al. The epigenetic landscape of oral squamous cell carcinoma. Br J Cancer 2013;108:370–9.

62. Kulkarni V, Saranath D. Concurrent hypermethylation of multiple regulatory genes in chewing tobacco associated oral squamous cell carcinomas and adjacent normal tissues. Oral Oncol 2004;40:145–53.

63. Kato K, Hara A, Kuno T, et al. Aberrant promoter hypermethylation of p16 and MGMT genes in oral squamous cell carcinomas and the surrounding normal mucosa. J Cancer Res Clin Oncol 2006;132:735–43.

64. von Zeidler SV, Miracca EC, Nagai MA, et al. Hypermethylation of the p16 gene in normal oral mucosa of smokers. Int J Mol Med 2004;14:807–11.

65. Yoo CB, Jones PA. Epigenetic therapy of cancer: past, present and future. Nat Rev Drug Discov 2006;5:37–50.

66. Smith IM, Mydlarz WK, Mithani SK, et al. DNA global hypomethylation in squamous cell head and neck cancer associated with smoking, alcohol consumption and stage. Int J Cancer 2007;121:1724–8.

67. Kurdistani SK. Histone modifications in cancer biology and prognosis. Prog Drug Res 2011;67:91–106.

68. Easwaran H, Tsai HC, Baylin SB. Cancer epigenetics: tumor heterogeneity, plasticity of stem-like states, and drug resistance. Mol Cell 2014;54:716–27.

69. Webber LP, Wagner VP, Curra M, et al. Hypoacetylation of acetyl-histone H3 (H3K9ac) as marker of poor prognosis in oral cancer. Histopathology 2017; 71:278–86.

70. Koshizuka K, Hanazawa T, Fukumoto I, et al. The microRNA signatures: aberrantly expressed microRNAs in head and neck squamous cell carcinoma. J Hum Genet 2017;62:3–13.

71. Lu J, Getz G, Miska EA, et al. MicroRNA expression profiles classify human cancers. Nature 2005;435:834–8.

72. Lajer CB, Nielsen FC, Friis-Hansen L, et al. Different miRNA signatures of oral and pharyngeal squamous cell carcinomas: a prospective translational study. Br J Cancer 2011;104:830–40.

73. Lagos-Quintana M, Rauhut R, Lendeckel W, et al. Identification of novel genes coding for small expressed RNAs. Science 2001;294:853–8.

74. Bartel DP. MicroRNAs: genomics, biogenesis, mechanism, and function. Cell 2004;116:281–97.

75. Gorenchtein M, Poh CF, Saini R, et al. MicroRNAs in an oral cancer context - from basic biology to clinical utility. J Dent Res 2012;91:440-6.

76. Friedman RC, Farh KK, Burge CB, et al. Most mammalian mRNAs are conserved targets of microRNAs. Genome Res 2009;19:92-105.

77. Liu S, Liu L, Ye W, et al. High vimentin expression associated with lymph node metastasis and predicated a poor prognosis in oral squamous cell carcinoma. Sci Rep 2016;6:38834.

78. Ye X, Weinberg RA. Epithelial-mesenchymal plasticity: a central regulator of cancer progression. Trends Cell Biol 2015;25:675-86.

79. Yan TL, Wang M, Xu Z, et al. Up-regulation of syncytin-1 contributes to TNF-alpha-enhanced fusion between OSCC and HUVECs partly via Wnt/beta-catenin-dependent pathway. Sci Rep 2017;7:40983.

80. Curry JM, Sprandio J, Cognetti D, et al. Tumor microenvironment in head and neck squamous cell carcinoma. Semin Oncol 2014;41:217-34.

81. Hino M, Kamo M, Saito D, et al. Transforming growth factor-beta1 induces invasion ability of HSC-4 human oral squamous cell carcinoma cells through the Slug/Wnt-5b/MMP-10 signalling axis. J Biochem 2016;159:631-40.

82. Medici D, Hay ED, Olsen BR. Snail and slug promote epithelial-mesenchymal transition through beta-catenin-T-cell factor-4-dependent expression of transforming growth factor-beta3. Mol Biol Cell 2008;19:4875-87.

83. Bagordakis E, Sawazaki-Calone I, Macedo CC, et al. Secretome profiling of oral squamous cell carcinoma-associated fibroblasts reveals organization and disassembly of extracellular matrix and collagen metabolic process signatures. Tumour Biol 2016;37:9045-57.

84. Gandellini P, Andriani F, Merlino G, et al. Complexity in the tumour microenvironment: cancer associated fibroblast gene expression patterns identify both common and unique features of tumour-stroma crosstalk across cancer types. Semin Cancer Biol 2015;35:96-106.

85. Lin NN, Wang P, Zhao D, et al. Significance of oral cancer-associated fibroblasts in angiogenesis, lymphangiogenesis, and tumor invasion in oral squamous cell carcinoma. J Oral Pathol Med 2017;46:21-30.

86. Cirillo N, Hassona Y, Celentano A, et al. Cancer-associated fibroblasts regulate keratinocyte cell-cell adhesion via TGF-beta-dependent pathways in genotype-specific oral cancer. Carcinogenesis 2017;38:76-85.

87. Takahashi H, Sakakura K, Kudo T, et al. Cancer-associated fibroblasts promote an immunosuppressive microenvironment through the induction and accumulation of protumoral macrophages. Oncotarget 2017;8:8633-47.

88. Fujii N, Shomori K, Shiomi T, et al. Cancer-associated fibroblasts and CD163-positive macrophages in oral squamous cell carcinoma: their clinicopathological and prognostic significance. J Oral Pathol Med 2012;41:444-51.

89. Zhang X, Li L, Wei D, et al. Moving cancer diagnostics from bench to bedside. Trends Biotechnol 2007;25:166-73.

90. Wang X, Kaczor-Urbanowicz KE, Wong DT. Salivary biomarkers in cancer detection. Med Oncol 2017;34:7.

91. Kim DH, Kim YS, Son NI, et al. Recent omics technologies and their emerging applications for personalised medicine. IET Syst Biol 2017;11:87-98.

92. Chin L, Andersen JN, Futreal PA. Cancer genomics: from discovery science to personalized medicine. Nat Med 2011;17:297-303.

93. Cancer Genome Atlas Network. Comprehensive genomic characterization of head and neck squamous cell carcinomas. Nature 2015;517:576-82.

94. Stein LD, Knoppers BM, Campbell P, et al. Data analysis: create a cloud commons. Nature 2015;523:149–51.
95. Wiklund ED, Gao S, Hulf T, et al. MicroRNA alterations and associated aberrant DNA methylation patterns across multiple sample types in oral squamous cell carcinoma. PLoS One 2011;6:e27840.
96. Tang H, Wu Z, Zhang J, et al. Salivary lncRNA as a potential marker for oral squamous cell carcinoma diagnosis. Mol Med Rep 2013;7:761–6.
97. Severino P, Alvares AM, Michaluart P Jr, et al. Global gene expression profiling of oral cavity cancers suggests molecular heterogeneity within anatomic subsites. BMC Res Notes 2008;1:113.
98. Walter V, Yin X, Wilkerson MD, et al. Molecular subtypes in head and neck cancer exhibit distinct patterns of chromosomal gain and loss of canonical cancer genes. PLoS One 2013;8:e56823.
99. Chung CH, Parker JS, Karaca G, et al. Molecular classification of head and neck squamous cell carcinomas using patterns of gene expression. Cancer Cell 2004;5:489–500.
100. van Hooff SR, Leusink FK, Roepman P, et al. Validation of a gene expression signature for assessment of lymph node metastasis in oral squamous cell carcinoma. J Clin Oncol 2012;30:4104–10.
101. He Y, Shao F, Pi W, et al. Largescale transcriptomics analysis suggests overexpression of BGH3, MMP9 and PDIA3 in oral squamous cell carcinoma. PLoS One 2016;11:e0146530.
102. Schwanhausser B, Busse D, Li N, et al. Global quantification of mammalian gene expression control. Nature 2011;473:337–42.
103. Malik UU, Zarina S, Pennington SR. Oral squamous cell carcinoma: key clinical questions, biomarker discovery, and the role of proteomics. Arch Oral Biol 2016; 63:53–65.
104. Lo WY, Lai CC, Hua CH, et al. S100A8 is identified as a biomarker of HPV18-infected oral squamous cell carcinomas by suppression subtraction hybridization, clinical proteomics analysis, and immunohistochemistry staining. J Proteome Res 2007;6:2143–51.
105. Hu S, Wong DT. Oral cancer proteomics. Curr Opin Mol Ther 2007;9:467–76.
106. Schaaij-Visser TB, Brakenhoff RH, Leemans CR, et al. Protein biomarker discovery for head and neck cancer. J Proteomics 2010;73:1790–803.
107. Wadsworth JT, Somers KD, Stack BC Jr, et al. Identification of patients with head and neck cancer using serum protein profiles. Arch Otolaryngol Head Neck Surg 2004;130:98–104.
108. Wang J, Christison TT, Misuno K, et al. Metabolomic profiling of anionic metabolites in head and neck cancer cells by capillary ion chromatography with orbitrap mass spectrometry. Anal Chem 2014;86:5116–24.
109. Yonezawa K, Nishiumi S, Kitamoto-Matsuda J, et al. Serum and tissue metabolomics of head and neck cancer. Cancer Genomics Proteomics 2013;10:233–8.
110. Hu S, Wang J, Ji EH, et al. Targeted metabolomic analysis of head and neck cancer cells using high performance ion chromatography coupled with a Q exactive HF mass spectrometer. Anal Chem 2015;87:6371–9.
111. Tie G, Yan J, Khair L, et al. Hypercholesterolemia increases colorectal cancer incidence by reducing production of NKT and gammadelta T Cells from hematopoietic stem cells. Cancer Res 2017;77:2351–62.
112. Codini M, Cataldi S, Lazzarini A, et al. Why high cholesterol levels help hematological malignancies: role of nuclear lipid microdomains. Lipids Health Dis 2016; 15:4.

113. Acharya S, Rai P, Hallikeri K, et al. Serum lipid profile in oral squamous cell carcinoma: alterations and association with some clinicopathological parameters and tobacco use. Int J Oral Maxillofac Surg 2016;45:713–20.

114. Patel PS, Shah MH, Jha FP, et al. Alterations in plasma lipid profile patterns in head and neck cancer and oral precancerous conditions. Indian J Cancer 2004;41:25–31.

115. Tran B, Dancey JE, Kamel-Reid S, et al. Cancer genomics: technology, discovery, and translation. J Clin Oncol 2012;30:647–60.

116. Tonella L, Giannoccaro M, Alfieri S, et al. Gene expression signatures for head and neck cancer patient stratification: are results ready for clinical application? Curr Treat Options Oncol 2017;18:32.

117. Stratton MR, Campbell PJ, Futreal PA. The cancer genome. Nature 2009;458:719–24.

118. Mardis ER, Wilson RK. Cancer genome sequencing: a review. Hum Mol Genet 2009;18:R163–8.

119. Gonzalez-Angulo AM, Hennessy BT, Mills GB. Future of personalized medicine in oncology: a systems biology approach. J Clin Oncol 2010;28:2777–83.

120. Razzouk S. Translational genomics and head and neck cancer: toward precision medicine. Clin Genet 2014;86:412–21.

121. Fabsitz RR, McGuire A, Sharp RR, et al. Ethical and practical guidelines for reporting genetic research results to study participants: updated guidelines from a National Heart, Lung, and Blood Institute working group. Circ Cardiovasc Genet 2010;3:574–80.

Printed and bound by CPI Group (UK) Ltd, Croydon, CR0 4YY

03/10/2024

01040406-0015